AYURVEDA

The Most Complete and Detailed Guide to
Ayurvedic Self Healing

(Natural Herbs Benefits for Healthy Living)

Craig Otoole

Published by Knowledge Icons

Craig Otoole

All Rights Reserved

Ayurveda: The Most Complete and Detailed Guide to Ayurvedic Self Healing (Natural Herbs Benefits for Healthy Living)

ISBN 978-1-990084-82-9

All rights reserved. No part of this guide may be reproduced in any form without permission in writing from the publisher except in the case of brief quotations embodied in critical articles or reviews.

Legal & Disclaimer

The information contained in this book is not designed to replace or take the place of any form of medicine or professional medical advice. The information in this book has been provided for educational and entertainment purposes only.

The information contained in this book has been compiled from sources deemed reliable, and it is accurate to the best of the Author's knowledge; however, the Author cannot guarantee its accuracy and validity and cannot be held liable for any errors or omissions. Changes are periodically made to this book. You must consult your doctor or get professional medical advice before using any of the suggested remedies, techniques, or information in this book.

Upon using the information contained in this book, you agree to hold harmless the Author from and against any damages, costs, and expenses, including any legal fees potentially resulting from the application of any of the information provided by this guide. This disclaimer applies to any damages or injury caused by the use and application, whether directly or indirectly, of any advice or information presented, whether for breach of contract, tort, negligence, personal injury, criminal intent, or under any other cause of action.

You agree to accept all risks of using the information presented inside this book. You need to consult a professional medical practitioner in order to ensure you are both able and healthy enough to participate in this program.

TABLE OF CONTENTS

INTRODUCTION 1

CHAPTER 1: PRINCIPLES OF AYURVEDA 5

CHAPTER 2: AYURVEDA DIETARY TIPS FOR A HEALTHIER SKIN 13

CHAPTER 3: PLANNING FOR WEIGHT LOSS? 17

CHAPTER 4: DANDRUFF 28

CHAPTER 5: AYURVEDA USES THE FIVE ELEMENT THEORY PANCHA MAHABHUTAS 36

CHAPTER 6: Ayurnedic Medicines And Important Herbs 45

CHAPTER 7: AYURVEDA: YOUR BODY AND PRAKHRITI 57

CHAPTER 8: WHO SHOULD PRACTICE AYURVEDA AND WHY? 70

CHAPTER 9: LOSING WEIGHT THROUGH AYURVEDA 78

CHAPTER 10: AYURVEDIC SECRETS FOR EXCELLENT DIGESTION 87

CHAPTER 11: HOW TO EXAMINE YOURSELF AND AVOID DISEASES 96

CHAPTER 12: SORE NIPPLES 104

CHAPTER 13: AYURVEDIC MEDICINE 112

CHAPTER 14: BALANCING VATA DOŞA WILL BALANCE ALL THREE DOŞAS 118

CHAPTER 15: SPARSHAN PAREEKSHA- BY HEARTBEAT ANALYSIS (AN OVERVIEW) 136

CHAPTER 16: ASHWAGANDA 165

CONCLUSION 170

Introduction

The Ayurveda is a form of alternative and complementary medicine (CAM). With the help of Ayurveda medication, you can achieve good health by achieving harmony of your spirit, body, and mind with this universe.

Any disruption in the balance may result in sickness and poor health. Numerous things can cause disruption, such as birth or genetic defects, seasonal and climate changes, age, emotions, injuries, etc. A unique constitution (parkriti) of your body is made of your unique psychological and physical characteristics. Your body composition remains same for your whole life, and it can affect different functions of your body. Every person in consist of five elements of the universe, such as space, fire, air, earth, and water.

These features make three energies or forces of life called doshas. Three doshas are Pitta dosha (fire & water), Vata dosha (space & air) and Kapha dosha (water & earth). These three doshas play an important role to control your body and one dosha typically remain dominant in each person. Every dosha is responsible for controlling various functions of the body, and your sickness chances are linked with the balance of these doshas.

Vata Dosha

The air and space dosha is considered a powerful dosha among all doshas. It controls the basic functions of your body, such as division of cells, breathing, mind, blood flow, ability to flush body waste out through your intestines and heart functions. Different things can affect this dosha, such as dry fruits, fear, overeating, grief and staying up late night. If this dosha is your main force of life, you may develop asthma, anxiety, heart disease, rheumatoid arthritis, skin problems and nervous system ailments.

Pitta Dosha

The water and fire dosha plays an important role to control your metabolism, digestion and particular hormones linked with appetite. Spicy and sour foods, fatigue and excessive exposure to the sun can disturb this dosha. If it is your fundamental life force, you may develop negative and anger emotions, Crohn's disease, heartburn after eating, hypertension, infections, etc.

Kapha Dosha

The earth and water dosha controls your weight, stability and body strength, muscle growth and immune system. Overeating, daytime sleeping, flavored drinks and food items, salty water, excessive consumption of sweet food and greed can disturb this dosha. If your main force of life is Kapha dosha, you may develop cancer, breathing disorders, nausea, asthma, obesity, diabetes and nausea after having a meal.

In this book, you will find some good recipes to make your herbal medications and treat numerous health problems.

Chapter 1: Principles Of Ayurveda

Concepts And Fundamental Principles

Most of the principles and fundamental theories of Ayurveda are based on experience and practice. Fourfold examination has ascertained them over the years – 1) authoritative statement; 2) perception; 3) inference and 4) rationale. Ayurvedic principle believes that the human body and the entire universe are one and governed by same principles. The changes witnessed by the universe, as the time passes, are also effective on the human body.

The universe and the human body both are believed to be made up of five constituent elements – the balanced state of which brings in good health while an imbalance causes disease. Ayurvedic medication aims to bring in such equilibrium in order to attain good health and longevity.

The concepts of pathology, physiology, diagnosis, medicine and therapeutics are based on the doctrine of tridoshas – vata, pitta and kapha. These doshas have the capacity to vitiate various other doshas as they are present in every human cell and keep moving through every channel in the body. In normal state, these doshas being main supports of the body are associated with different functions. Vata governs the activities of the nervous system; pitta is responsible for thermogenic and endocrine/exocrine glandular activities; and kapha governs the muscoskeletal and anabolic systems.

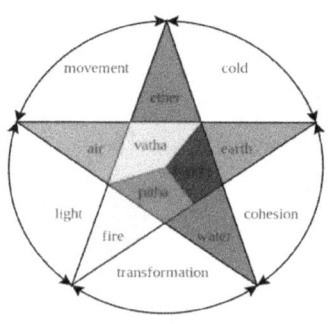

The three *doshas* and the five elements they are composed of

Then there are seven dhatus – the basic tissues of the human body which also act as support. The seven dhatus are: 1) rakta (blood); 2) rasa (nutritive elements which make up the end product of digestion); 3) mamsa (muscle tissue); 4) medas (adipose tissue); 5) asthi (cartilage and osseous tissue); 6) majja (red bone marrow); and 7) shukra (reproductive elements).

Then, comes the third important element – mala – the main excretory wastes of the body like mutra (urine), purisha (faeces) and sveda (sweat).

Ayurveda aims to maintain equilibrium between the three elements dosha, dhatu and mala.

Ayurvedic Pharmacology

Ayurvedic medicines are made up of substance of natural origin including parts of animals, whole or parts of plants and minerals used in combination or alone. These medicines and the ayurvedic processes work on the principles of vishesha (antagonistic) and samanya (homologous) action. To increase the elemental properties or constituents in the body, substances with homologous properties are used while vishesha is used to decrease those constituents. All the processes work with an aim to restore balance among dosha, dhatu and mala.

The action of medicines depends on various properties which are considered to study the composition of various constituents of a medicine. These properties are:

a) Rasa (taste) – it is a property of medicine which is detected by tongue. The six tastes are salty, sweet, pungent, sour, astringent and bitter.

b) Guna – 20 in number, these are those characteristics of a medicine which are detected by sense organs other than tongue. Some examples of it are: heavy/light; dull/sharp; hot/cold, etc.

c) Virya – divided into two broad categories, virya denotes the potency of a medicine. The two broad categories are: sita (cooling) and ushna (heating).

d) Vipaka – it establishes the state of rasas after digestion as demonstrated by their action.

e) Prabhava – when a medicine cannot be explained by its elemental composition that special property is called as prabhav.

Ayurvedic Pathology

Ayurveda recognizes three main causes of any disease:

a) Indiscriminate use of senses and their objects.

b) Error of intellect which results in loss of differentiation between wholesome and unwholesome with consequence indulgence in unwholesome diets and behaviour.

c) Effects of time, seasonal variation and cosmic effects.

Diagnosis is based on five components of pathology of disease – 1) causative factors; 2) prodromal symptoms; 3) signs and symptoms; 4) pathogenesis and 5) elements antagonistic to disease and causes.

There are six stages of pathogenesis that help in understanding the occurrence of a disease. These are 1) accumulation; 2) aggravation; 3) overflowing; 4) localization; 5) manifestation and 6) classification or dissolution.

Treatment of a disease comprises of three main ways – 1) avoidance of causative and provocative factors; 2) purifying therapies and 3) palliative therapies.

Ayurveda has 8 elements of diagnosis – 1) Nadi (pulse); 2) Mootra (urine); 3) Mala (stool); 4) Jihva (tongue); 5) Shabda (speech); 6) Sparsha (touch); 7) Druk (vision); and 8) Aakruti (appearance).

AYURVEDIC THERAPEUTICS

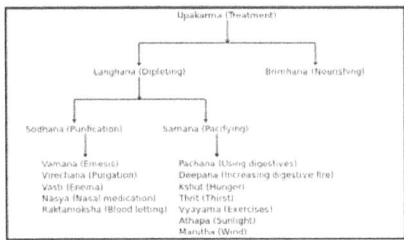

Ayurveda works to preserve equilibrium of dhatus in healthy individuals in order to prevent diseases. Once the disease is set in, the treatment eliminates the imbalance between the doshas and thereby restores the body to normality. Keeping in view the point that the ultimate aim is to maintain equilibrium in all individuals, the wholesome substance is divided into two types – one that maintains health and two that alleviates the disorders by correcting the abnormal doshas. First one acts in healthy people while the second one is important for diseased people.

Some of the prescribed ayurvedic therapeutic measures are as follows:

a) Promoting body weight.

b) Producing lightness in the body.

c) Diaphoretic.

d) Roughening.

e) Proper purification by elimination of impurities.

f) Food

g) Behaviour and conduct.

Out of 8, only two branches of classical ayurveda deal with surgical treatment. Contemporary ayurvedic theories lay stress on building a attaining good digestion, healthy metabolic system and proper excretion. Other than this, ayurveda also focuses on meditation, yoga and exercise; importance of natural cycles like walking, sleeping, working, etc; maintenance of hygiene, bathing, cleaning teeth, skin care, and eye washing.

Chapter 2: Ayurveda Dietary Tips For A Healthier Skin

Taking care of your skin is a great way to maintain your physical appearance. In addition, skin is the largest organ of your body. Thus proper maintenance is needed in order to make the skin function well. Unfortunately, most of us don't realize that skin health is important until some problems occur. Pimples, blemishes or spots are some problems that commonly occur on your face skin. These problems happen due to diet disorders or certain lifestyle. If you select a more skin friendly diet, then these problems may not occur.

Ayurveda, the oldest healthcare system, can be your ideal choice in improving skin's health. Ayurvedic science helps people prevent diseases through meditation, herbs, nutrition and daily routines. To help you take good care of your skin, Ayurveda has some dietary tips for you. Below are the tips you can apply:

1. Lemon

Lemon is good for your skin since it is able to flush out toxins in your body. Thus your skin will stay clean and fresh. You can make juice of half a lemon and mix it with a glass of hot water. This beverage should be consumed in the morning. For those with oily skin, they can have another glass of lemon water in the afternoon or evening.

2. Herb Tea

Herb tea is one of the most important parts in ayurvedic skin care. You can have various flavors of tea such as cardamom, cinnamon, aniseed or mint. To get the best result, you should take it twice or thrice a day. Some herbs that work well to clean your skin are Sarsaparilla, marshmallow root, turmeric and Indian madder. They purify your blood and clean toxins in the body.

3. Raw Salads

Raw salads can be an ideal choice for your health. However, you can obtain the maximum benefit of raw food only when your digestive system is strong enough. If you don't have a strong digestive system, you will find difficulties in digesting the food. Ayurvedic skin care suggests that you consume vegetables with high water content. Some vegetables that are good for your skin are lettuce, tender asparagus and carrots. In Ayurvedic science, these vegetables are called as tridoshic. It means that they are suitable for any skin types. You can also have cruciferous vegetables to improve your skin's health. However, these vegetables should be steamed first as they are difficult to digest.

A complete Ayurvedic skin care recommends you to avoid taking oily foods and bad fats. Instead, you are recommended to increase your fresh food intake like vegetables and fruits. These Ayurvedic dietary tips will help you make a big difference in your skin without taking the costly treatments.

Chapter 3: Planning For Weight Loss?

You don't have to starve yourself to **lose weight**; in fact, you shouldn't. Losing weight the healthy way involves a commitment to your plan and patience. Appropriate planning is key for successful weight loss. Combining your weight loss plan with ways to control your **metabolism** can help you to reach your goal more quickly, and still lose your weight the healthy way.

Be sure you need to lose weight, and that this is the best time for you to proceed with weight loss. If you have a medical condition, your body may need added calories to maintain your health, so this is not the time to start losing weight. If you have medical conditions such as hypertension, diabetes, or cardiovascular problems, consult your doctor before starting a diet and exercise plan. Many factors, including age, current weight, and overall physical health, are relevant in order to safely start a diet and exercise plan.

Weight loss in a moderate way is a healthy approach. Allow yourself the time you need to reach your weight loss goal, planning on a reasonable loss each week. While it may be tempting to pursue fad diets with promises of fast weight loss, a slow and steady approach is the healthiest way to lose weight and Ayurveda is the one that offers that not as a treatment but as a life style. While fad diets may help you to drop weight quickly, they are not sustainable long term and once you stop the fad diet, you often gain back the weight plus more.

Weight loss happens when you burn more calories than you consume. It is highly recommended to determine the number of calories to consume each day specific to your body, age, sex, and your lifestyle.

One pound is equal to about 3,500 calories. In order to lose 1 to 2 pounds each week, your daily calorie consumption needs to decrease by about 500 to 1000 calories, or you activity level needs to increase to burn more calories. One has to avoid setting the daily calorie goal too low. This can actually prevent you from losing weight. When you skip meals or consume too few calories, your body starts to store calories as fat instead of burning them. However, don't starve yourself. Your body stores up more calories as fat, instead of burning them, when calorie intake is drastically reduced.

Reduce your use of alcoholic beverages. Alcohol contains a lot of calories. Stop drinking beverages with sugar. A glass of coke contains 8-10 teaspoons of sugar. Try water, tea, or black coffee. When exercising for the first time, don't overdo it. You are more likely to learn to enjoy exercising if you begin gradually. Healthy weight loss occurs at a steady pace. Remember that you are aiming for a permanent change, not a quick fix. Avoid eating right before bed. Eating late causes your body to store the food as body fat. Get your whole family involved in habits for healthy eating and lifestyle changes. This is a healthy choice for everybody.

Come and join the Ayurvedic lifestyle which gives you a plan that fits your own likes and dislikes. Many healthy weight loss plans already exist and can be tweaked to suit your own preferences and needs. Whether you tweak a formal diet plan or come up with your own, be sure it is suited to you, and is a plan you can live with for a long time, not just for a few months. This is where ayurveda gains importance by offering a lifestyle than a treatment. As you are aware, a life style offers you a lifetime remedy. For a successful healthy lifestyle change, it is important that your new plan fit into your life without too much difficulty. Adjusting how you eat and exercise is one thing, completely changing to foods you don't normally eat and exercises you don't enjoy will most likely not be successful in the long term.

As you develop your plan, incorporate what worked, and leave out what did not work. Add your own personal preferences, and include flexibility in both your food and physical activity choices. Plus, consider your preference to diet all alone. Remember there is a cost for everything. Similar cost applies for a slimmer you as well in the form of club membership fee, protein supplements, diet alternatives etc.

Successful weight loss requires a commitment to yourself to stick with your plan for the long term. Some people find it helpful to put your plan in writing. Include why you want to lose the weight, the plan itself, how much weight you want to lose, and your target date to reach your desired weight. Then sign it as if you are signing a contract.

The cost of being slim

Six-pack abs, tight butts, slim, vibrant, flawless health. This is the image the fitness industry is selling. But have you ever wondered what it costs to achieve that "look"? What you really have to give up? Make no mistake, there are real trade-offs as you attempt to lose fat and improve your health. Let's talk about what they are. So you can consider how to get the body you really want while living the life you really enjoy.

It is a misconception that with just a few small, easy, hopefully imperceptible changes to one's diet and exercise routine, you too can have shredded abs, big biceps, and tight glutes. On the other hand it is also not true that getting into shape involves painful, intolerable sacrifice, restriction, and deprivation. The reality is that the first 10 pounds is not the same one that will help you lose "the last 10 pounds". Indeed, it usually takes a lot more work as you get slimmer. If you do aspire to "fitness model" or "elite athlete" slim, you might be surprised. Images are photoshopped for effect. Bodybuilders only look like that for competition. And achieving that look comes at a high cost; one most people aren't willing to pay.

However, if you're okay not being on the next magazine cover and aspire to be "slim and healthy" even small adjustments can over time add up to noticeable improvements. Sometimes these improvements can change, perhaps even save, lives. Maybe you pack an apple in your lunch instead of apple juice. Or you include a salad with dinner, or you stick to one or two drinks with friends. And you're feeling good! Your knees have stopped hurting, plus your pants now button comfortably. Now you're somewhere in the zone of "a little extra padding, but not too bad". You're more mobile, healthier, and high-fiving yourself.

Elite bodybuilders getting ready for a contest and models getting ready for a shoot are basically in a slow starvation process. Adhering to an extremely strict and precise regimen of eating and training is the only way they can drop their body fat to extremely low levels. It goes against biological cues. It requires exercising when exhausted. It demands ignoring their desire for food in the face of powerful hunger cues. It involves intense focus and dedication. And it often distracts from other areas of life that these athletes might enjoy and value.

You have to make your own food and measure every meal down to the last gram. That food is generally very plain - slim protein, steamed vegetables, plain potatoes or rice, etc. You can't think straight because you're always hungry and tired. Your whole life revolves around making food, dieting, training, and recovery protocols. Is that level of slimness worth it? Having a six-pack doesn't automatically make you healthy. In fact, getting too slim can be actively unhealthy. In short, being really slim has almost nothing to do with being really healthy. Indeed, being too focused on getting slim may lead you away from good health. Some folks have staggered abdominals. Some have angled abdominals. Some people might really only have four abdominals that are visible no matter how slim they get.

Whatever change you want to make, remember: It will take time. Eating one big, rich meal won't make you wake up overweight. Fasting for 24 hours won't give you six-pack abs. A simple plan followed consistently is better than a complex plan followed intermittently. You'll have to put in more time and more effort. Plus, you'll need to follow your plan even more consistently with almost obsessive accuracy.

From "slim" to "slimmer"

You need to do the following stuff:

a. Get more exercise and daily-life movement and make that exercise more intense

b. Eat more vegetables and slim protein

c. Choose more whole foods

d. Do your meal plan – preferably 5 a day

e. Be serious about rest

f. learn your hunger and fullness cues

Try to avoid or at least reduce the following stuffs:

drinking alcohol and other high-calorie beverages

eating processed foods

eating when you're not physically hungry

You have to make these small changes consistently, over a period of time. It is vital that you have recognized the fact that in order to change, you have to change. At super slim stage, going from athletically slim to bodybuilder slim, the tradeoffs get even more serious.

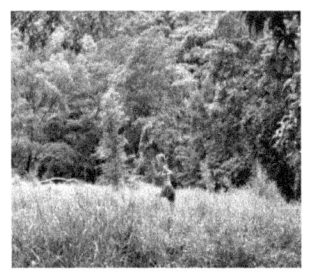

Chapter 4: Dandruff

Dandruff is one of the most common scalp disorders wherein accumulation of dead skin cells appears onto the scalp in the form of white flakes. This flaky layer of dead cells gets in the way of free breathing of your hair and thus weakens it, leaving it more susceptible to fall out. Furthermore, these scales fall onto the shoulders, eyebrows and even clothes when you comb or scratch your scalp. Therefore, those affected always feel conscious in the crowd.

Dandruff might be the result of a number of factors such as frequent heat or cold exposure, excessive exposure to hair styling products, chronic constipation, stress, fatigue, pollution and much more. There are lots of shampoos that boast of clearing white flakes, but most really fail to do so. Let's take the ayurvedic route to get rid of dandruff. There's no harm in trying these ayurvedic remedies for dandruff, you never know it might just work wonders for your hair.

1. Camphor with coconut oil:

This is one of the grand maa's recipes where you just need to mix small amount of camphor in coconut oil. Store it in a bottle, and apply each night before going to bed. Camphor cools your scalp and helps to reduce dandruff.

2. Coconut with lemon:

Lemon is a key ingredient in most of the hair care remedies. Mix lemon in warm coconut oil and apply on the scalp. Leave it for about half an hour before shampoo. Follow this for at least two weeks for best results.

3. Gram flour with curd:

Mix two spoons of gram flour in a small bowl of curd. Add half a spoon of lemon juice. Apply this mixture on your scalp and leave it for thirty minutes. Curd and gram flour are best hair cleansers that aid in cleaning the scalp. This definitely the best ayurvedic medicine for dandruff to try.

4. Curd with lemon:

Ayurvedic remedies for dandruff are many but this is one that has lasted the tested of time. Just a bowl of curd with two lemons squeezed in it is one of the best ayurvedic remedies to get a clean and clear scalp. Lemons are supposed to be real dandruff killers. It is worth trying this tip. Curd acts as a moisturizer and keep your scalp cool.

5. Shikakayee Concoction:

Mix Shikakayee with mint leaves and fenugreek seeds. Soak them in water and apply the mixture on the scalp before you sleep. Leave it overnight. In the morning, rinse it off with warm water. If you cannot prepare it at home, there are many ayurvedic shops that sell already packed shikakyee with many more herbs great for the hair.

6. Neem leaves with lemon

Make a paste of neem leaves. Add half a lemon to it and apply the paste onto your scalp. Leave it for 30 minutes and wash it with shampoo. For best results, use this tip twice a week.

7. Hot oil massage:

Before you apply any oil on your hair, just warm it up a little for the oil to get soaked deeper in the roots. Massage your hair with hot oil before going to bed.

8. Almond oil with Olive oil:

Mix almond oil with olive oil. Both are known to have superb qualities to help your hair grow as well as nourish it. Make sugar solution and apply it on your hair after the oil massage. After the shampoo, use tea water to rinse at last.

9. Vinegar ayurvedic remedy:

Mix two tablespoons of vinegar in cup of hot water. Use cotton to dab on the scalp. Vinegar not only conditions your hair but also assists in clearing dandruff.

10. Mint leaves with apple cider vinegar:

Boil a cup of water mixed with a cup of apple cider vinegar. Add few mint leaves. Let the mixture boil for some time and allow it to cool. Gently take the mixture on your finger tips and massage it into your scalp. Rinse after it dries.

11. Sandalwood Oil:

Another version of Ayurveda treatment for dandruff comes in the form of sandalwood oil-lime juice mixture. The emulsion should be massaged onto the scalp for a few minutes and then washed out with tepid water. Massage treatment will boost circulation, strengthen hair roots and improve the overall health of your hair apart from remedying dandruff.

12. Amla Paste:

A simple anti-dandruff hair pack created with Amla powder, Tulsi leaves and water works wonders to cure this pesky and irritating hair condition. One must rub this paste onto the head thoroughly and let it sit for almost 30 minutes. As soon as the set time is over, rinse hair with plain water.

13. Aloe Vera:

The thick gel extracted from Aloe Vera leaves is a putative remedy for coping dandruff-related issues. Simply spread the gel all over your hair and leave overnight. Shampoo your hair as usual next morning.

14. Eggs:

Eggs are a powerhouse of several hair-benefiting nutrients and thus are considered extremely useful for the hair. A potion produced with egg and water works like magic to throw the dandruff away, if applied to the scalp regularly and rinsed out later on with fresh water.

15. Wheat Germ Oil:

Another fine way to get rid of dandruff is to deep condition the hair with wheat germ oil. First get a through head massage with warmed up wheat germ oil and then cover up the head with a clean towel. Don't forget to dip the towel in warm water so as to warm it up slightly. Also make sure to squeeze excess water before you wrap it around your head. Wait for about half an hour and then wash your hair off with water.

16. Black Pepper Powder:

Black pepper powder, blended with milk and fresh lime juice is known to provide a great solution for dandruff problems. The concoction is supposed to be rubbed onto the scalp thoroughly and then left on for an hour. Rinse out finally with plain water.

17. Fenugreek seeds:

Fenugreek seed paste, prepared by soaking the seeds in water overnight and mashing the next morning, is found to be highly beneficial in treating dandruff. Get the paste thoroughly applied onto your hair and scalp for 30-45 minutes and then rinse off. Besides being one of the best ayurvedic dandruff treatments, it is also very effective in curing hair loss.

Try these ayurvedic dandruff treatments and you will see why this type of treatment is more prefered to anything else!

Chapter 5: Ayurveda Uses The Five Element Theory Pancha Mahabhutas

Pancha Mahabhutas

The universe consists of different combinations of the five basic elements: earth, water, fire, air, and space. The Pancha (five) Mahabhutas theory classifies not only all earthly objects but also natural cycles like the seasons – spring, summer, autumn, and winter. It is a powerful system to understand how man interacts with his environment.

The five elements (mahabhutas) have attributes that impact your body and mind. All matter is a mixture of the five elements, but has one dominant element that defines it. The balance and nature of elements is never static - temperature (agni/ fire), dryness (vayu/ air), humidity (jala/water) etc. are in a natural state of flux. Severe weather can occur when this combination becomes volatile or extreme. That is when thunderstorms, hurricanes, floods or drought occurs.

Human Composition: Humans are one of the many living organisms on earth and are essentially made up of the same elements that form all of the other entities on earth. Death returns our bodies to the earth, water, fire, air and space. A person maintains the combination of elements already present in the body by respiration and nutrition - absorbing those elements found in the natural world. The "five element" theory explains the connection between humans and the rest of the natural world. Thus foods and herbs can help to heal the human body. Flora can repair and regenerate humans because they share an elemental basis.

Ayurveda creates two distinct classifications of a person; one relating to the body and the second to the mind. One's nature, or Prakriti, is determined by this combination of body and mind classifications.

Dosha specifically refers to three biological energies – kapha, pitta and vata. In Sanskrit, dosha is defined as "that which contaminates". Doshas are pathogens or disease-causing vectors. An imbalance of vata, pitta and kapha doshas cause disease in the body.

When there is imbalance in dosha illness occurs in the body. According to Ayurveda human body is segregated into these three body types. An ayurvedic practitioner will know which body type you belong to by looking at you as well as from the symptoms of your illnesses. For example if you're overweight, feel lazy, have sinus problem, chest congestion and your hair and skin is oily, you dislike cold weather then you're suffering from kapha dosha and you need to balance it.

The Sanskrit definition of a Guna is a characteristic, an influence or impulse. Knowing your Dosha and Guna gives an understanding of your basic physical and psychological nature. Knowing your prakriti/ nature helps you to tailor a personalized diet and lifestyle that can help prevent disease and physical disorders, to obtain peace of mind. This knowledge helps to maintain balance with your surroundings and that is the key to good health. Your elemental nature or dosha is unchangeable. However the mind can play a role in re-shaping your nature through acquiring positive qualities, and minimizing negative mental characteristics.

Three qualities - the Gunas: Guna may be defined as a characteristic or quality. A guna may also be an influence or impulse. All cosmic matter is said to be made up of three gunas. Just as your body contains all of the elements; your mind also has each of the gunas. The three basic gunas/qualities are: Sattva (knowledge, purity), Rajas (action, passion), and Tamas (inertia, ignorance).

In the human context, guna refers to the mental nature and personal character. Whether a person is sattvic: gentle, calm, tolerant and patient, or rajasic: greedy, passionate, impulsive, exploitative, materialistic and focused on sensual gratification, or tamasic: slothful, ignorant, deceitful and insensitive - is governed by the gunas.

As the mind is intimately connected with the body, increasing contact or consumption of rajasic or tamasic things creates an imbalance in the mind and distresses the body. This manifests as disease and illness in many forms. If a person's dosha is imbalanced it disrupts the mind guna.

Modern status: Ayurvedic physicians coalesced into professional associations in the 20th century. Ayurveda is now a statutory, recognized medical system of health care in India. CCIM - The Central Council of Indian Medicine - governs the system. Ayurveda practitioners in India undergo 5 1/2 years of studies and one year of internship in Ayurveda medical schools upon which they qualify for a professional doctorate degree called Bachelor of Ayurvedic Medicine and Surgery [B.A.M.S.].

Western Practice: Due to medical practice rules & regulations in the West, Ayurvedic treatments are commonly practiced as massage therapy and as dietary / herbal nutrition. The National Institute of Ayurvedic Medicine in the USA is an institute that carries out Ayurvedic research regularly.

As regards intellectual property rights - some western (US & European) pharmaceutical companies and academic institutions have conflicted with their Indian counterparts and traditional practitioners of Ayurveda over the IPR's of certain natural products newly researched in the West. Indian practitioners have known about the pharmacology of these products for centuries and thus claim precedence on their patent rights.

Criticisms - Scientific studies / standards: Primary criticisms relate to the lack of rigorous scientific studies or clinical trials of many ayurvedic products. The National Center for Complementary and Alternative Medicine states that "most clinical trials of Ayurvedic approaches have been small, had problems with research designs, lacked appropriate control groups, or had other issues that affected how meaningful the results were."

Safety issues: There is laboratory evidence that the use of certain ayurvedic medicines involving herbs, metals, minerals, and other materials results in serious toxicological and metabolic risks.

JAMA - the Journal of the American Medical Association - published a research study where it was found that significant levels of toxic heavy metals such as lead, mercury and arsenic exist in over 20% of Ayurvedic medicines made in South Asia for sale in the US. JAMA concluded that, if consumed according to the manufacturers' prescriptions, these substances "could result in heavy metal intakes above published regulatory standards". Similar studies conducted in India have confirmed this.

"Miracle Cures": critics also debate the safety of those Ayurvedic medicines that claim to be "Miracle Cures". This is because "miracles" are subject to theological rather than scientific inquiry.

Ayurvedic wisdom originated within the Vedas as a way of life - an intimate connection with nature and spirit. It then evolved into medical aspects which took priority over the spiritual forms of healing. As Ayurveda becomes globally commercial - its spiritual aspects may recede. However there is an increasing body of physicians who weave Ayurveda's spiritual therapies most effectively into the medical realm - with spectacular results.

Ayurvedic science and medicine is ancient, but continues to endure with a relevance and wisdom for human beings across the ages. It has offered curative hope to people and civilizations over centuries. Its gentle wisdom embraces an intimate knowledge of the spirit and its temple, the body. Today, scientific advances have finally begun to keep pace with this ancient healer of men.

Chapter 6: Ayurvedic Medicines And

Important Herbs

What is Ayurveda and Its Importance? Ayurveda is a traditional holistic healing. Translated from Sanskrit, Ayurveda means 'the science of life'. ayur means "life" and veda means "science. India system which largely depends on plant support to form major Chunk of its medicine. Most of the herbs, spices, seeds, roots, leaves, stems, petals and flowers are deeply ingrained in all Indian homes where 'home remedies' are popular. Even certain family members in some family are adept in curing even intricate disorders by simple and cost effective formulations which, at times, have shown marvelous and astounding results. All over the world today we are looking for a natural system of healing that is comprehensive and complete, that is not merely some curious form of folk healing but a real and rational system of medicine that is sensitive to both nature and the Earth.

This is exactly what Ayurveda has to offer, for it has a many thousand year-old clinical tradition and a comprehensive natural method of treatment ranging from diet, herbs and massage. With Ayurveda we learn the right diet for our individual type, how to improve our immune system, he keys to right use of sexual energy and rejuvenation,a nd a conscious way of life that can lift us to a new level of awareness in all our endeavors. Without such natural wisdom as Ayurveda, we may find ourselves not only unhealthy, but unhappy and spiritually confused. Ayurveda Principles and Theory Ayurveda system is the prominent user of herbs and its basic theory revolves round imbalance and vitiation of three humors (Doshas). Ether (Akash), Air (Vayu), Fire (Agni), Water (Jal) and Earth (Prithvi) are the great five elements which underline all living systems. these elements are constantly changing and interacting and can be simplified into three Vitiations (Doshas). When these doshas remain under harmony and balance, health of body does not get disturbed but, when their balance gets disturbed, a diseased state sets in.

The three doshas are vata (Wind), Pitta (Bile) and Kapha (Phlegm) and due to predominance of the one dosha, a person's personality is determined that is ' Vata- Prakriti', 'Pitta- Prakriti' or 'Kapha Prakriti' Vata formed from ether and air, governs all movement in the mind and body and must be kept in good balance. Pitta formed from fire and water, governs "all heat, metabolism and transformation in the mind and body Kapha formed from earth and water, cements the elements in the body, providing the material for physical structure. Each person has an individual blend of the three doshas, with one or sometimes two doshas predominating. Common Herbs used in

Ayurvedic Medicines Amalaki (Amla or Indian Gooseberry or Emblica officinalis) - The fruit is reputed to have the highest content of vitamin C of any natural occuring substance in nature. It maintains balance amongst three doshas and effectively controls digestive problems, strengthens heart, normalises cholesterol, prevents cancer, builds up and sustain defence mechanism, improves eye-sight and detoxifies the body. Amla is said to have 20 times more vitamin C than orange. The vitamin C content of amla is between 625mg - 1814mg per 100gms. Other studies show that amla increases red blood cell count and hemoglobin.

A research tem discovered that when Amla is taken regularly as a dietary supplement, it counteracts the toxic effects of prolonged exposure to environmental heavy metals, such as lead, aluminium and nickel. Read More About Amla http://www.ayurvediccure.com/amla.htm Ashwagandha (Winter Cherry or Withania

Somnifera)- Ashwagandha is one of the main herbs for promoting ojas and rejuvenating the body in Ayurveda. It is a well known semen promoter and it treats impotency and infertility. Clinical studies show that Ashwagandha has antibacterial, antitumor, anti-inflammatory and immunomodulating properties. The strong anti-stress actions, increases memory and learning capabilities. It has also found to be useful in Rheumatic and Arthritic disorders like pain, swelling etc Summing up, it is a strong Aphrodisiac and has Immunomodulating, anti- inflammatory, anti tumor and anti stress properties which clearly shows why Ayurveda has such a high opinion of this herb as a general tonic. Read More About Ashwagandha http://www.ayurvediccure.com/ashwagandha.htm Arjuna (Terminalia Arjuna) - It is a cardiac tonic of high quality. Terminalia arjuna, is known to be beneficial for the treatment of heart ailments since 500 BC. Clinical research has indicated its usefulness in relieving anginal pain, and in the treatment of coronary artery disease, heart failure, and possibly hypercholesterolemia. "Terminalia arjuna bark extract, 500 mg 8 hourly, given to patients with stable angina with provocable ischemia on treadmill exercise, led to improvement in clinical and treadmill exercise parameters as compared to placebo therapy."

Result on Clinical Research Conducted. Improvement of cardiac muscle function and subsequent improved pumping activity of the heart seem to be the primary benefits of Terminalia Arjuna. Read More About Arjuna http://www.ayurvedicure.com/arjuna.htm Brahmi (Bacopa, Gotu Kola) - Brahmi is known as "the food for brain". Traditionally Brahmi is used as a mental tonic, to rejuvenate the body, as a promoter of memory and as a nerve tonic. It promotes a calm, clear mind, and improves mental function. Modern

Research claims that brahmi improves memory and helps overcome the negative effects of stress. Brahmi is especially suitable for students as it enhances the minds ability to learn and to focus and for an elderly person hoping to regain their memory. It is unique in its ability to invigorate mental processes whilst reducing the effects of stress and nervous anxiety.

As a nervine tonic, Brahmi has been used to help those affected by stroke, nervous breakdown or exhaustion and Attention Deficit Disorder. The best Ayurvedic brain and memory formulas contain brahmi, as do many of the long life promoting compounds. Read More About Brahmi http://www.ayurvediccure.com/brahmi.htm Guggulu (Shuddha Guggulu, Guggul, Commiphora Mukul) - Modern Research shows that it is the prime Ayurvedic herb for treating obesity and high cholesterol. Studies shows that guggulu lowers serum cholesterol and phospholipids, and that it also protects against cholesterol- induced atherosclerosis. Guggulu were seen to lower body weight in these clinical studies. Guggulu also as anti-inflammatory properties and is effective in treating arthritis and other joint pains. Read More About Guggulu http://www.ayurvediccure.com/guggul.htm Karela (Bitter Melon, Bitter Gourd, Momordica Charantia) - At least three different groups of constituents have been reported to have blood sugar lowering actions in bitter Mellon.

These include a mixture of steroidal saponins known as charantin, insulin-like peptides, and alkaloids. Scientific studies have consistently shown that bitter melon lowers blood sugar level of Type 2 Diabetes. It could probably reduce the patients intake of antidiabetic drugs. Also Bitter Melon has two proteins which are thought to repress the AIDS virus. Recently, the Department of Health in the Philippines has recommended bitter melon as one of the best herbal medicines for diabetic management. Read More About Bitter Melon http://www.ayurvediccure.com/bittergourd.htm Neem (Azadirachta Indica) - Neem is an extraordinary blood purifier, good for al skin diseases like acne, eczema, psoriasis and teeth and gums. Neem is included in most Ayurvedic Skin products because it is as effective on an external application as through internal indigestion. In Ayurveda it has been safely used for over five thousand years and are a good immunity booster to prevent colds, fevers, infections and various skin diseases. Read More About Neem http://www.ayurvediccure.com/neem.htm Shilajit (Mineral Pitch, Asphaltum) - Shilajit is one of the prime Ayurvedic compounds for rejuvenating the body. it is an aphrodisiac, anti-aging herb and to treat diabetes and debilitating urinary problems. The Charaka Samhita states that a person must use shilajit for a minimum of one month before starting to realize he regenerating effects. It is also used to treat impotency and infertility. it is well known that Shilajit would return the libido of people to level of teenagers. There is a folk saying by the indigenous people who live in the Himalayan region that Shilajit makes the body strong as a rock. It is an adaptogen, (Rasayna), that helps to combat immune disorders, urinary tract disorders, nervous disorders and sexual dissatisfaction. Read More About Shilajit http://www.ayurvediccure.com/shilajit.ht m Shallaki (Boswellia Serrata, Salai Guggul) - Modern Research indicate that the Boswellia herb may assist in treating joint mobility, pain, and may be a useful remedy for a variety of inflammatory diseases like rheumatoid arthritis and osteoarthritis.

A recent clinical trial suggests positive effects of Boswellia serrata extract in knee osteoarthritis. Boswellia has also been found to be useful for a number of other disorders and best for treating Back Pain, Knee Pain, Joint Pain and Arthritis. This herb has also been proposed as a possible therapy for Crohn's disease and ulcerative colitis. Read More About Boswellia http://www.ayurvediccure.com/shallaki.htm Triphala (Amalaki, Bibhitaki, Haritaki) - Triphala has got the properties of three famous nutrients: amla, haritaki and bibhitaki. The advantage of this formula is that it is milder in action and more balanced than any of the three alone. It has cleansing and detoxifying action. Used regularly it is good for gentle, slow detoxification of the digestive tract and then the deep tissues. It also has the ability to normalize all three humors with continued use. As a daily supplement triphala is hard to beat; that' s why in India they say "even if your mother leaves you, every thing will be fine if you have triphala" Read More About Triphala http://www.ayurvediccure.com/triphala.htm Tulsi (Holy Basil, Ocimum Sanctum) - Its very name Holy Basil certifies to its sacred nature. It is a sacred plant worshipped in many Indian homes and is a must in every Hindu's house. Holy basil is also a major ingredient of many Ayurvedic cough syrups. it is a good stress reliever, and modern research has found it to be good for Respiratory problems, Cold, Fever and all types of Cough. Read More About Tulsi. http://www.ayurvediccure.com/tulasi.htm

Chapter 7: Ayurveda: Your Body And

Prakhriti

Prakhriti/Dosha/Body Type

Your Ayurvedic body type is your heredity. Your genetics.

These qualities are dictated by the proportion of Doshas in the constitution of your mother and father, and the season in which conception happened, the goal/perspective and general prosperity of your parents.

This is the reason Ayurveda underscores over and over the significance of arranged conception, that both parents are healthy and of complimentary Doshas to ensure the best possible chance for a healthy offspring.

After conception happens, the nourishment from the mother to the embryo must focus on quality and building the growing fetuses constitution. For example, if the mother lives in a manner of prosperity, with proper nourishment and calming exercise, the child will be of sound constitution and an in-born protection from infection. If the pregnant mother eats a poor diet and takes no part in an exercise regime, the baby will be conceived with a weaker constitution and will have more difficulties.

Exercises for your Dosha

Our bodies are intended for physical movement—it is crucial to enjoying a life of vitality. Indeed, getting regular activity is one of the most effective things you can do to stay strong, limber, and stave off the aging process.

According to Ayurveda, activity should be suited to one's Dosha. Each Dosha lends itself to certain activities.

Let's assume somebody is exceptionally Kapha. They're laid back and don't enjoy strenuous activity, yet they have great stamina; it would be right to propose a long, lively walk. In contrasts, Vata types have high energy levels, but if they are overweight, a slower and more relaxed walk would be most beneficial. Pitta sorts fall some place in the center and benefit from moderate activity.

KAPHA

Kapha Doshas have solid, relentless vitality and incredible physicality. They are adept at exceeding expectations in endurance sports like long distance running, high impact exercise, soccer, paddling, etc. Any sort of aerobic exercise that works up a decent sweat is effective for clearing Kapha blockages and motivating them.

On the off-chance that you are Kapha dominant, your greatest test may be discovering the inspiration to work out. In the event that you have not been active for some time, you can break the habit with energetic walking, starting with 30 minutes at a time.

To feel an observable change, it is vital to work up a sweat. You may need to wear a two-layer activity outfit, for example, an all-cotton sweat suit under a nylon suit. Bit by bit expand your activity to incorporate running, hiking and bicycling.

Exercises for this Dosha

Weight lifting

Running

Treadmill

Cardio

Speed walking

Elliptical

PITTA

Pitta sorts tend to like competitive activities, for example, skiing, climbing, tennis, and mountain climbing. Due to their focused nature, Pittas need to be mindful so as not to build their anxiety while exercising, stewing over every terrible golf shot or needing to win no matter what.

If you are a Pitta, you might particularly appreciate winter sports because you can tolerate the cold better than Kaphas and Vatas. Pittas have a tendency to have less perseverance than Kaphas yet are great at resistance activities. You may also enjoy long-distance bicycling or rollerblading. Swimming is also a perfect activity for Pitta Dosha. The water cools the warmth of Pitta and mitigates the collected strain of the day.

Exercises for this Dosha

Softball

Tennis

Baseball

Swimming

Diving

Other water sports (i.e., water polo)

Note: Avoid the sun.

VATA

Vata type have bursts of vitality and a tendency to tire rapidly. In the event that they are out of balance, Vatas are especially inclined to pushing themselves too hard.

Vatas benefit tremendously from grounding activities, for example, yoga, simple walks and leisurely bicycling. These exercises help Vata Doshas develop badly needed equilibrium. In the winter, indoor activity is suggested for Vatas because they hate the cold and often don't have enough fat and muscle to keep them warm.

It cannot be said enough: choosing activities suited to your psyche and body type will give you the best results and contentment. You are more likely to sustain the activity if you are well-suited to it.

Regardless of what your present wellness level is, the key is to move your body and relax. Add exercise to your normal routine and you will enjoy invaluable vitality and satisfaction.

Exercises for this Dosha

Yoga

Pilates

Walking

Moving

Weights

Improv dance

Ballet

Ayurveda—Incorporating it into your diet

The biggest change you can make right now to your diet would be to start drinking room temperature or warm water rather than ice water. There is nothing that destroys the digestive flame (agni) faster than ice water on an empty stomach.

Knowing which tastes and qualities are best for your Ayurveda Body Type will help you to settle on the right choices, whether eating out or preparing food at home.

For instance, for Vata, warm soup is a better choice than a chilled mixed green salad. Because Vata adapts best to warm and is upset by cold. When eating out, stay far from raw, cold dishes and concentrate on well-cooked, warm dishes.

In the event that you have a dominant Pitta Dosha, you are best served by having a cold meal such as a raw vegetable platter. Avoid broiled foods, and anything with garlic or tomato because hot and spicy foods irritate Pitta.

If Kapha is your prevailing Dosha, you will do best with light choices, such as steamed vegetables. Stay away from dishes that are greasy or laden with heavy cheese sauces.

Ayurveda acknowledges that there are six tastes and it's vital to have these in your eating routine consistently. The six tastes are:

Sweet

Sugar

Syrup

Rice

Pasta

Milk

sour

Citrus

Cheddar

Yogurt

Vinegar

Salty

Black olives

Peppers

Cayenne

Fresh ginger

Pungent

Hot peppers

Onions

Garlic

Salts

bitter

Dark greens

Turmeric

Dandelion root

Astringent

Pomegranate

Beans

Broccoli and cauliflower

Lentils

These six tastes are noted in the order in which they are processed in your body. Sweet gets processed first, making the habit of having dessert last unhealthy for our bodies. Similarly, in conflict with what we have been trained to accept, salad should be had at the end of your meal. The Ayurveda Diet has an exceptionally through diet routine.

Ensuring that each of the six tastes are included in your meal aids in feeling fulfilled. Cravings are thought to be triggered by not having the six tastes in your daily diet. The bitter and astringent tastes are the most lacking. Yet, when you have something sharp or astringent toward the end of a meal, it actually eliminates the need or want for dessert.

Losing weight with the help of Ayurveda

The concept of the "ama" in Ayurveda is critical to getting in shape. "Ama" is defined as "toxins." They are the sticky waste product left after digestion and when not dealt with properly, pollute our bodies and literally make us sick. They are the consequence of inappropriate diets, endless anxiety and environmental toxins. Some of these poisons are water-soluble, making them less demanding to expel from the body with proper diet and activity. However, some are fat-soluble, wherein they get settle inside fat cells. The fat cells extend as they absorb these toxins, causing weight gain particularly in those difficult to lose pockets of fat around the stomach, hips and thighs.

Ayurvedic methods work on expelling ama from your body, which in turn shrinks your fat cells. With proper detox programs to help evacuate the build-up then a good maintenance plan according to your Dosha, you can find balance.

The fundamental guidelines

One of the biggest hurdles when it comes to weight loss has to be eating irregularly and particularly having large meals late at night. As Ayurveda shows, our metabolism is slowed at night, and when we sleep, our digestion and absorption slow drastically. The body basically can't process large, late night suppers efficiently. The outcome is a significant part of the nutrition is inadequately digested and ultimately becomes toxins, fat and excess weight.

Hot water with ginger or lemon or herbal teas consumed as often as possible throughout the day can help you improve your digestion considerably. Drinking hot water frequently over the day aids to purify your digestive tract and clear many blockages. Hot water enhances nutrient absorption; an added bonus is that it reduces cravings and hunger pangs between meals. This in turn reduces the desire for overly processed prepared snacks.

One unique belief of Ayurveda is that food loses its nutrients as it chills in a fridge or when reheated as a leftover. The emphasis must be on freshly prepared foods in order to get the greatest health pay-off.

Important to ensuring proper digestive functions and key to the mind/body connection lauded by Ayurveda, you need to find five to 10 or more minutes of peace and solitude in the morning. Mind/body practices like yoga, meditation or qi gong promote a relaxation response in the body. This serves to assuage stress, one of the fundamental drivers of weight gain. It additionally places us in a more mindful and present place in our brain, allowing us to be better people as our day unfolds.

Chapter 8: Who Should Practice Ayurveda

And Why?

Can Ayurveda Cure Existing Illnesse or Just Redress Doshic Imbalances?

Ayurveda should be practiced by anyone who needs some improvement in their life. If you experience health problems, Ayurveda can help you regulate the areas of your body that are affected by alternative means while also addressing your emotional health, your mental energy, and your general outlook.

One of the first steps when you visit an Ayurvedic practitioner will be spotting your dosha and seeing what potential imbalances may lead to certain health problems or imperfect state of mind. For instance, you may suffer from flatulence or other digestive problems because your diet doesn't include the right nutrients to balance your doshic constitution. Or you may simply be too apathetic, lethargic, or slow because one dosha is lacking from your personality (e.g. Pitta). In such cases, Ayurvedic theories and practices can help you regain your balance and your happiness.

You don't have to have a serious health problem to include Ayurveda in your life. It's enough if you don't feel completely satisfied with yourself or you don't experience life to the fullest for some obscure reasons. Doshic imbalance may manifest itself subtly and surreptitiously sometimes. Do you feel you don't have enough appetite? Do you have panic attacks? Have you experienced too many mood swings lately? Are you unfulfilled in your romantic life? Do you feel emotionally labile? Do you wish you were more competitive and driven? Would you like to be able to focus better and be more creative in your professional life instead of methodical and linear?

Such cases are only a few examples of "problems" that you may experience quite strongly or only vaguely. In any case, Ayurveda can help you encourage what you miss or what you crave in your life. If you just don't feel happy enough, you are easily distracted, you feel you're getting too introverted and alienated from the world and other people, or you can't relax as you should, you should try resorting to Ayurveda to manage any imbalance that these problems may be based on.

Needless to say, you are totally welcome to practice Ayurveda and regulate your doshic constitution when you experience mild to serious health problems that can be easily tracked down to a highly "inflated" dosha or lacking energy. For instance, too much nervous energy, flakiness, and loss of interest after the initial stages of a project/relationships signal a Vata imbalance. Inertia, excessive resistance to change, and too much dependence on routines is a clear sign of too much Kapha. Skin eruptions or irregular and abnormal stools indicate you should balance out your Pitta. Any such situations from simple digestive problems to asthma, joint pain, or rheumatism can be treated by means of Ayurveda. Even more severe conditions e.g auto-immune diseases are likely to be cured after systematic and consistent Ayurveda practice and the corresponding changes in overall lifestyle and mental outlook.

Why should you start practicing Ayurveda? Simply put, this source of ancient wisdom provides you with extra tools to combat unwanted issues in your body and your life. Of course, if you are experiencing severe health problems, you should also consult a medical specialist apart from including these alternative medical practices in your life. More often than not, Ayurvedic medicine doesn't negate classic medicine. The point of adopting Ayurveda in your life is enhancing the treatment you receive in such a case and benefitting from additional tools to ensure recovery and well-being.

A Holistic Approach to Your Health and Wellbeing

Keep in mind that Ayurveda starts from a holistic approach to health. Thus you will not only be addressing, say, your digestive problems, but you'll also reach a state of improved energy and increased happiness by practicing Ayurveda. The remedies you will use if you practice Ayurveda are not expensive at all and extremely natural. You will be including many plants and herbs in your diet in order to manage any imbalance you may go through.

What more can you ask for? This will bring you closer to the power of nature and to the life force that flows through everything that surrounds you. Ayurvedic treatment has absolutely no side effects. You run no risk and you have nothing to lose, especially if you use Ayurveda as an alternative to classic medicine when you have a severe health problem. You should know however that Ayurveda has proven quite efficient in treating rather complicated issues such as chronic diseases, immunity imbalances, or mental problems.

Ayurveda is also a great weapon against potential problems you may face as you grow older. Even if you don't suffer from anything specific and serious issues, but you feel you would like to enjoy more energy and vitality in your overall activities or to simply adopt a more healthy diet, Ayurveda can help you reach your goal and improve your life. Ayurveda is great if you only want to prevent disease. It keeps your body, your mind, and your energy fields healthy and pure. Ayurveda is also amazingly beneficial when you go through periods of intense strain due to work pressure or exams at school. It can help you focus better, improve your memory as well as your performance, and simply feel more revitalized and driven in everything you do. Instead of resorting to B-complex and Lecithin supplements in such stressful situations, how about starting to practice Ayurveda? It is the best means of balancing your body and stimulating your mind to achieve what you want and reach your whole (even latent) potential.

Ayurveda can be used for both specific health problems that can be traced back to certain organs or functions in the body and a visible improvement of your overall emotional and mental state. At the same time, given its strong connection to ancient Hindu philosophy and wisdom, Ayurveda can also help you find your path in life or the meaning you crave if you feel you are uprooted, confused, or devoid of a sense of deeper significance. Remember that Ayurveda can also act as a spiritual catalyst and guide in case you feel you lack such a force or dimension in your life. If you are disappointed with what the religious systems you're already familiar with can offer you, try tapping into Ayurvedic wisdom. If you feel you are not certain about your beliefs and you simply lack a center that can offer you stability and hope, Ayurveda can help you discover many interesting things about life and yourself that you may otherwise totally ignore. We live in a world in which the commercial and the technological have too much of a say sometimes. This can make us feel our lives risk becoming empty, mechanized, or meaningless. Ayurveda can help you connect to a valuable source of ancient wisdom that has guided many people along centuries.

Chapter 9: Losing Weight Through Ayurveda

Mind and body balance in the Ayurveda diet take precedence over weight loss. However, if you want to lose weight through Ayurveda, know that you are overweight probably because your kapha dosha is not balanced. It's also important to know that your body has the three dosha types, with one or two dominating others. In Ayurveda, the kapha dosha may be helped through dietary intervention.

Ayurveda claims that individuals prone to the kapha dosha have low digestive fire, and they should do away with consuming heavy meals. People having low digestive fire should consume lighter meals, instead. Those who are predominantly kapha should limit eating sour, salty and sweet foods that call for high digestive fire to digest.

If you are predominantly kapha, increase your intake of pungent, astringent or bitter foods that promote digestive enzyme secretion. Consuming cold foods and beverages may aggravate the kapha dosha. Kapha people should not also eat too quickly or too slowly. Eating at a high or slow pace may prompt a person to overeat.

Excess in Kapha Dosha

In Ayurveda, being overweight entails an excess of kapha dosha. While it may not be the sole factor in dealing with excess weight, kapha certainly plays an important role. One of Ayurveda's main principles is that opposites balance and like increases like.

Excess weight and kapha have similar attributes. Both of them slow, heavy, smooth, oily, cool, soft, dense, gross and stable, thus, being overweight can provoke the body's kapha. Excess body kapha can lead to obesity. On the contrary, achieving balance entails a surge in opposing influences like sharp, light, dry, hot, liquid, rough, subtle and mobile.

The Ayurveda diet does not center on short-term gains, so you don't need to starve yourself deliberately, or limit the food variety you can enjoy unrealistically. With the Ayurveda diet, you can follow a time-tested and clear path to excellent health.

When you are trying to lose weight through the Ayurveda diet, you may consider committing to follow five simple steps to help you reach your desired weight.

Do yoga for 15 minutes every morning.

Eat three satiating meals every day.

Adhere to a kapha pacifying diet.

Exercise for a minimum of three days a week.

Set a daily routine to support your weight loss commitments.

The commitments are intuitive and simple. While you may have to exercise discipline in the beginning, your body's inherent intelligence will soon resurface with balanced urges in place of unhealthy cravings. When you attain such balance, sticking to your commitments gets easier until you notice that they are already becoming second nature.

One of the book's important topics is losing weight through the Ayurveda diet. Below are pointers on following the kapha pacifying diet. As mentioned earlier, an excess of kapha leads to obesity. If you feel that you are overweight, you may have to know more about the kapha pacifying diet.

Kapha Pacifying Diet

Kapha balance is attained by eating a diet rich in whole, freshly-cooked foods that are dry, light, well-spiced, relatively easily digestible and warming. Such foods are best served hot or warm. The foods normalize kapha by regulating moisture levels, balancing mucus production, maintaining sufficient heat and supporting elimination and proper digestion.

As kapha is naturally substantive, the right diet is one of the most efficient ways to achieve your desired weight. Kapha calls for a minimalistic diet with small quantities, fewer sweets, little snacking or none, various legumes, an abundance of fresh vegetables and fruits and minimal to no alcohol.

Qualities to Avoid and Favor

Kapha is smooth, oily, cool and heavy. Eating foods to neutralize kapha qualities (foods that are rough, dry, warm and light) can help to normalize kapha.

Favor airy and light over heavy and dense. Vegetables and fruit are light, thus, a diet based on fresh fruits and vegetables (cooked) is a great way to begin the kapha pacifying diet. Kapha is also balanced by raw vegetables and salads when they are in season. Black and green teas are preferable over the heavier coffee.

In general, avoid heavy foods like puddings, hard cheeses, cakes, nuts, wheat, pies, pastas, bread, most flours, deep fried foods, and red meat. Overeating at one sitting also causes heaviness. Avoid processed foods and heavy meals as they aggravate kapha's heaviness.

Favor warm over cold or cool. Eat foods with a warming energy. This means you need to utilize heating spices. Fortunately, spices are naturally warming and nearly all of them balance the kapha. Cooked foods are easily digestible and offer a warmer energy. Especially during the colder months, drink only hot, warm, or room temperature beverages. Conversely, avoid cooling energetic foods, frozen and cold drinks or food, leftovers from the refrigerator, and carbonated drinks.

Favor dry over oily or moist. The oiliness of kapha is offset by drying foods like popcorn, rice cakes, dried fruits, white potatoes, beans, and the rare glass of white or red wine. When cooking, use oil sparingly. You also need to minimize or eliminate foods like coconut, avocado, buttermilk, olives, eggs, cheese, cow's milk, eggs, nuts, seeds, and wheat. Kapha can easily retain water, so you must not drink water or liquids to excess. Moreover, avoid moist foods like summer squash, melons, yogurt, and zucchini, all of which can provoke kapha.

Favor rough over smooth. Vegetables and fruits' fibrous structure lends them a rough quality. Vegetables and fruits are easily digestible when cooked, but you should avoid overcooking them. Certain foods like cauliflower, cabbage, broccoli, many beansand dark leafy greens are high in roughage and can counteract kapha's oily, smooth nature. However, eating smooth foods like rice pudding, bananas, milk, hot cereal and cheese, can rapidly aggravate kapha.

Tastes to Avoid and Favor

Kapha is aggravated by the salty, sour and sweet tastes and is pacified by the bitter, astringent and pungent tastes. Understanding the tastes enables you to navigate the diet without constantly referring to lists of foods to avoid and favor.

Remember to emphasize pungent, bitter and astringent tastes. Minimize or avoid sweet, sour and salty tastes.

Eating to Balance Kapha

How you eat can impact your success when it comes to pacifying kapha. To balance kapha, you may want to eat three meals daily and eat those meals consistently. There are others who say that two meals are sufficient. You can also jumpstart a slow digestive fire (agni) for about 30 minutes before dinner and lunch by chewing ginger with a few lime juice drops, a pinch of salt, and ¼ teaspoon honey.

Excess bread, sweets and fast food can provoke kapha. You can lessen such foods' detrimental potential by ensuring they are served warm, taken sparingly, and are seasoned with warming spices and herbs. As kapha digestion is somewhat sluggish, you can also benefit with periodic cleanses or fasts. A short juice or fruit fast or a kichari monofast may help in the weight loss process.

Chapter 10: Ayurvedic Secrets For Excellent Digestion

Today, majority of the people in the world notably in America, suffer from severe indigestion problems such as gas, bloating, weakness after eating, burning, and pain in the stomach and heart burn. Ayurveda simply portrays simple methods and methodologies to solve all these issues. Ayuvreda attaches special importance to the process of digestion and considers digestion to contribute greatly to the physical heath of a person. Indigestion can cause great difficulty and a sense of being too uncomfortable. Ayuvreda from its origins from India, has emerged as a great solution for the solution of these problems.

There are a few secrets of ayurveda and some excellent tips which are as follows:

11. Commence your meal with some fresh ginger and a tiny bit of salt

Ginger is an ayuvredic herb which is known for its property of aiding in the digestion process. This ginger is an excellent help for those who suffer from problems like constipation, and those whose taste buds do not recognize the taste of the food. In other words, tastelessness!

Ginger is also a natural remedy for the cure of cough, cold and flu issues. For people who have inflammation problems or stinging should however avoid ginger. Salt plays a great role in the process of digestion. The role of the salt is that it stimulates the enzymes in the mouth which leads the tongue to eventually activate its taste buds. With activated taste buds a person is more likely to taste their food better. For much better digestion, hydrochloric acid plays a very important role and it is salt which makes this acid. The lining of the stomach walls is done by the hydrochloric acid. The secretion of this acid aids greatly in the digestion process. Eventually, salt is a great agent that helps the body in digesting its food.

12. Have warm water as a drink and warm food

Studies have proven that those eating their drink and food while warm do not face any indigestion complications. About it they say that the warm food and drink relates to the fire in the ayuvreda concept. The example related with it defines that like any substance which is cold if thrown in the fire extinguishes it so similarly when we eat cold food and drink it makes the fire to disappear thus slowing the digestion process or else diminishing it completely. On the other hand, when eating warm foods and warm drinks these then automatically initiates the the digestion process. This is why ayuvreda recommends consuming warm foods and drinks.

13. Cherish every eating experience to be very sacred on all times

Ayuvreda commands a lot of respect regarding the food on the plate when placed before a person. There is vast amount of knowledge in the ayuvreda concept about treating your meal as worthy of being sacred. It points out to take outgood quality time before every meal time, have a lot of respect, realize that getting a full plate of food actually means a person should thank God for the blessings and feel a rush of gratitude and to cherish the moment.

According to ayuvreda, it refuses to accept the way people have developed their eating habits to be today. For instance, sitting on the sofa, with the plate held delicately in hand, watching your favourite television show along with it or else using your smart phones along with eating. Ayuvreda suggests that following these methods the digestion process is a lot more different and perhaps not that effective also.

The latest technology of today, no matter very advanced and easy in this difficult world, has lead to many serious problems as well. The concept of eating together with the whole family, talking and listening to each other's problems has long gone. People prefer to eat along with their mobile phones or the television. Ayuvreda suggests that by considering the food to be sacred gives people the time to think about their food carefully, and to recognize the tastes it has and also makes the food to be chewed really slow rather then very fast in a illiterate manner, eventually aiding up in effective digestion.

14. To sit on the knees post dinner, yoga

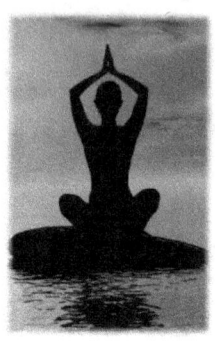

The term sacred eating also refers to ones behaviour after their dinner. Ayuvreda suggests to give the stomach a good amount of rest after your meal and not to run fast around the whole house. It does so by sitting in a form of yogic pose called Vajrasana, which is a position involving the hips to rest on the heels and both toes to be connected with each other and sitting on your knees.

Yoga is a great part of the ayuvreda concept, so to follow this means to help one own self in their digestion systems. If one is unable to sit in this exact Vajrasana pose, it will still help just if one will stand up straight and close their eyes for some minutes simply in memory of the food they have just had. This thought will ultimately give energy and nourishment to the mind and body.

15. The recommendation to cook with ayuvredic spices which aid greatly in digestion

There are numerous ayuvredic spices, all of which can be added in to the food cooked. And of course all of these spices play a vital role in speeding up the digestion process. Examples of these ayuvredic spices are ajwain seeds, fenugreek seeds, cumin seeds and asafetida. These all spices can be added to the meals and each of them has digestive properties which greatly aid in the digestion process.

Apart from digesting the food, these spices also help in preventing gas and bloating in individuals. These two problems cause a real sense of problem and can be excruciatingly painful at times. Gas and bloating is also caused when a person continuously eats and snacks, for instance without giving the necessary time to let adjust one meal or snack, they start eating up again. Adequate amount of time should be given to each meal to let it digest before eating again. Eating when hungry gives a real sense of comfort, energy and body also feels light.

16. Staying away from food when emotions are on a high level

In this topic, ayurveda comments that there is a link which connects food and emotions and both if not properly digested can lead to problems. If a person is emotionally disturbed, is in anxiety, is angry, in grief, depression he/she must not eat at that time. It is advisable therefore to calm your nerves and be normal before starting your food.

Ayuvreda believes that eating food when emotions are at high level can really heat up the digestion process. Even normally apart from ayuvreda, when a person is angry or when the emotions high it is very hard to compose. In that situation a person may eat up a lot more then needed or else eat in the wrong manner.

All these secrets were some ayurvedas principles of aiding in excellent digestion methods. Follow these and feel a real change in your body.

17. Ayuvreda also mentions to eat your meal in a peaceful and subtle environment for better digestion.

18. Ayuvreda suggests eating a piece of ginger before the meal or some pomegranate puree,

19. Drink lassi with or before your meal.

20. Avoid fizzy drinks and ice cold water during or after the meal.

21. Ayuvreda suggests having a hearty lunch and a light dinner.

Chapter 11: How To Examine Yourself And Avoid Diseases

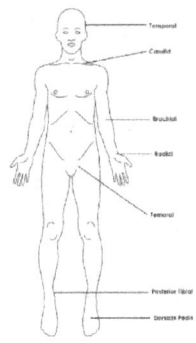

Usually, people go to their doctors to be examined after particular symptoms start manifesting or when they feel really sick. The procedure most likely will be as follows: symptoms – diagnosis –treatment – follow up. However, in Ayurveda, the diagnosis may be defined as the continuous at the moment interactions between the doshas and the bodily tissues. This is because it is believed that this is how disease manifests itself.

A daily observation, awareness and monitoring of the radial pulse, tongue, skin, etc is a very effective practice when it comes to disease prevention and also is a tool for self diagnosis. The following are guidelines that will serve as aid in the diagnosis and prevention of diseases:

Examination of the radial pulse –there are seven pulse points as seen in the diagram above. They are the temporal (above the temple), carotid (side of the neck above the clavicle), brachial (inside of the arm, above the elbow), radial (on the wrist), femoral (on the inside front of the leg), posterior tibial (behind the ankle) and dorsalispedis (top of the foot). .One of them, the radial pulse found at one's wrist in one's bodyis a good diagnostic point to at least have an idea on the state of one's body.

It is important to note that one's pulse should not be monitored after these events as one may get different or above normal results: while hungry, while taking a bath, after consummation, after taking food or alcohol, after hard physical labor, after massage and after urination. It is best to monitor one's pulse in the morning, after waking up or during times when one relaxed, rested and not at the peak of an emotional turmoil.

The status of the body organs and one's constitution can be identified when one is knowledgeable in the examination of radial pulse. The beats that one feels in pulsation not only indicates the beating of the heart but also gives an overview in the important meridians that connects pranic currents inside the body.

When doing an examination of the pulse, know that each finger rests on a meridian that corresponds to a particular body organ. To illustrate, the index finger gives an indication of the status of the lungs, the middle finger, of the intestines and the ring finger, of the kidneys. Making it a habit to check one's pulse and the changes that happens to it is an effective technique in self diagnosis.

Facial diagnosis — the face can be considered a mirror of the soul, thus diseases, at most times, reveal their ugly heads in one's face. Each line or spot in one's face can be an indication of what is going on inside one's body. Eyebrows, especially those with vertical lines may indicate repressed emotions are being stored in the liver. In the forehead, horizontal wrinkling could mean anxiety attacks and deep-seated worries. Whereas, a vertical line between the eyebrows may mean that the spleen is holding a lot of negative emotions. The kidneys may indicate impairment through dark and puffy eyes.

A discolored cheeks and nose may indicate something is wrong in one's kidneys and that the body is lacking folic acid and iron.

In general, based on constitutions, a Vata person does not have the ability to store fat so his face may look sunken and his nose crooked. A Kapha tends to accumulate water and most of the time has a puffy face and a blunt nose. A Pitta tends to have a good appetite and his face may look plump while his nose, sharp.

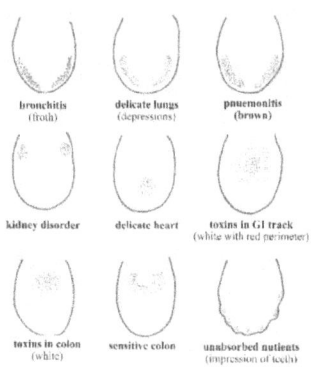

Tongue diagnosis – the tongue is the organ for taste and speech. It is vital for speech as it is integral to form sounds and makes it possible to convey ideas, feelings, thoughts and concepts. When the tongue is wet, it is able to perceive taste, when it is dry, it loses its ability to do so. It is important to make it a habit to check one's tongue as it reveals a lot of what's happening inside the body. The factors to consider when examining the tongue are the following: shape, color, size, margins, dampness and color.

The color yellowish may indicate bile in the gallbladder or liver disorder. It paleness is observed, problems in the blood may be considered. If the tongue is bluish and one has not eaten anything of bluish color, the heart ailment may be present. Teeth impressions in the tongue indicate intestinal disorders. Usually, coated tongues are indications of toxin overload in the body. Moreover, if one has observed a line in the middle which is quite impressed. It may indicate that emotions are being suppressed while a curved line may mean a spinal problem

Lip diagnosis - lips that are rough and chapped usually indicates dehydration and signals problems in the Vata dosha. Tremours and shaking of the lips may indicate anxiety attacks and nervousness. Pale lips are usually an indication of anemia or problems in the blood. Brown spots in the lips may indicate worms or may be a result of smoking habits. It is also important to note that Vata lips have a tendency to be thin and dry, Pitta lips are red and plump while Kapha lips are often thick and oily. The organs most associated with the lips are the internal organs, lungs, intestines, thyroid and the heart.

Eye diagnosis – round, big and beautiful eyes are of the Kapha constitution. Small, slanted, and those that blink constantly are Vata constitution. The Pitta eyes are usually sensitive to light and are lustrous to look at. A dropping eyelid may indicate a feeling of insecurity and lack of self-confidence to the beholder. Prominent eyes usually are a sign of hormonal imbalance or a dysfunction in the thyroid gland. In case one observes a white ring around the iris, it is an indication of too much salt or sugar in the body. Spots in the eye, especially those that are colored brown indicate nutrients that are not absorbed in the body.

Nail diagnosis – the Ayurveda principle believes that the nails are a waste product of the bones. The factors to consider when examining the nails are the following factors: contour, shape, size, color and surface. It also helps to observe whether the nails are brittle, soft, breaks easily or if they are even-colored. Vata constitution usually has nails that are crooked, breaks easily and are rough to hold. Pitta nails are soft, pink or light-colored and have a tendency to glisten.

Chapter 12: Sore Nipples

- Sore nipples is a common problem faced by new mothers
- The condition can make it difficult for a woman to breastfeed

Symptoms to look for:

- Cracked and painful nipples

Causes:

- Yeast infection
- Improper feeding position makes it difficult for the baby to suck milk and results in tearing of nipples

Natural home remedy using basil leaves:

1. Crush a handful of basil leaves to make paste
2. Apply this paste on the affected area
3. Wash off before the feeding session
4. Do this several times a day

Natural home remedy using ice:

1. Take a few ice cubes

2. Wrap them in a clean piece of cloth

3. Place this on the affected area for 2-3 min

4. Repeat this 3 times a day

Natural home remedy using aloe vera:

1. Take a few aloe vera leaves

2. Remove the thorns and the outer skin

3. Extract its gel from inside

4. Apply this gel on the nipples

5. Make sure to wash it off before the next feeding session

Endometriosis:

- Endometriosis is a common health disorder affecting women
- The condition can cause problems in conceiving

Symptoms to look for:

- Painful periods
- Painful cramps during menstruation
- Pain in the lower abdomen
- Pain during sexual intercourse

- Painful bowel movement

Causes:

- Certain cells, which are supposed to grow in the womb lining, start to grow outside the uterus, leading to this condition

Natural home remedy using milk and asparagus powder:

1. Take 1 glass of warm milk
2. Add 2 tsp of Indian asparagus powder
3. Mix well
4. Drink 2 times a day

Natural home remedy using the Ashoka tree's bark:

1. Crush the bark of an Ashoka tree to powder, commonly available at ayurvedic stores
2. Take 2 tbsp of this powder
3. Mix it in 250 ml of water
4. Heat this water till only half the liquid remains
5. Strain the liquid

6. Drink 2 times a day

Natural home remedy using flax seeds:

1. Take 4 tbsp of flax seeds

2. Soak them in 1 cup of water overnight

3. Strain and drink this water the next morning

Tips:

- Drink pineapple juice to quicken the healing process

Morning Sickness:

- Morning sickness affects pregnant women in the 6th and 12th week of pregnancy

- Contrary to what the name suggests, the symptoms of this condition can occur anytime during the day

Symptoms to look for:

- Nausea
- Vomiting
- Dehydration

Causes:

- Rise of estrogen levels in the body
- Imbalance of electrolytes and glucose

Natural home remedy using curry leaves, lemon juice and sugar:

1. Crush a handful of curry leaves
2. Press them on a sieve and extract their juice
3. Take 2 tsp curry leave juice
4. Add 1 tsp lemon juice
5. You may add sugar for taste
6. Mix well
7. Drink 2 times every day

Natural home remedy using mint leaves, ginger, lemons and honey:

1. Take 1 tsp mint leaves' juice
2. Add ½ tsp ginger paste
3. Add 1 tsp lemon juice
4. Add 1 tsp honey
5. Mix well
6. Drink 2 times every day

Natural home remedy using mint leaves:

1. Take a handful of mint leaves

2. Boil them in 200 ml water

3. Inhale the fumes for relief from morning sickness

Tips:

• Do not get up from the bed immediately after sleep - wake up slowly

• Keep biscuits or crackers handy for early morning snacks

• Eat multiple small meals through the day

• Avoid fried, oily and spicy foods

• Avoid alcohol and caffeine intake

Mastitis:

• Mastitis is a bacterial infection of the breast tissue

• New mothers develop mastitis during breastfeeding

• Bacteria enters the breast through the cracks present in the nipples

• The condition causes pain which hampers the breastfeeding process

Symptoms to look for:

- Around the breast:
  o Pain
  o Warmth
  o Redness
  o Swelling
- Fever
- Chills

Natural home remedy using cabbage leaves:

1. Take a few cold cabbage leaves
2. Press them on the breast
3. Replace the leaves when they reach room temperature

Natural home remedy using fenugreek seeds:

1. Soak 3-4 tbsp fenugreek seeds in water overnight
2. Crush them to a paste in the morning
3. Apply this paste on the breast
4. Leave it for 15 min
5. Cover it with a cloth

6. Repeat 2 times a day

Tips:

• New mothers should wear lose clothes, which do not cause any discomfort or friction around the

nipples

Chapter 13: Ayurvedic Medicine

The Ayurvedic medicines are itself is called as ayurveda. In Sanskrit language 'Ayu' is the term for life and 'veda' for the science. Hence, Ayurveda means studying the science of the life.

Benefits Of Turning To Ayurveda or Ayurvedic Medicines

No side effects -the most important benefit of taking ayurvedic medicines is that generally consuming them would have no side effects.

No chemicals – Unlike other medicines, basically the ayurvedic medicines would not have any chemicals in their medicines. The ayurvedic medicines are made from the natural herbal products.

Could be continued with other therapies too – Having ayurvedic medicines would not make you stop at adopting the usual therapies that one takes for curing an ailment.

Proven to be beneficial – It is stated that ayurveda was prevalent since 1500 B.C. Hence from the times immemorial it has been tried and tested and many major serious diseases like asthma, diabetes, heart diseases have been cured with the help of ayurvedic medicines.

Medicines:

oConstitutents of ayurvedic medicines:Almost all the medicines used in treating diseases or ailments in ayurveda comprise of just naturally cultivated herbs. One or more herbs with some other natural ingredients are mixed together to form a curable preparation for any specific ailment.

o Other components: Ayurveda advocates lifestyle changes and diet control for almost all the problems that a human being would be suffering from. Other than the herbs which have medicinal properties, ayurvedic medicines comprise of some flowers, fruits, along with the common kitchen herbs and other vegetation.

The common factor in all the medicines of ayurveda is that they would comprise of only natural vegetation. With no chemicals or toxins involved.

The ayurvedic medicines would generally comprise of:

Powders, Oils that are medicated, Decoctions etc

Treatment:

Ayurveda its stated that, has been prevalent since 1500BC. Its effectiveness should be understood from its prevalence itself. Ayurvedic medicines treat the diseases from its root cause.Therefore, the treatment in ayurveda itself is deep rooted.

Each disease would have a different kind of approach, for each individual.However, ayurveda categories human body into 3 types. The first one is vata body type and then pitta and kapha.

Body Types:

The 3 body types mentioned above could be combined into minimum of 10 possible combinations which are as follows:

 "Vata" ayurvedic body type have in them the air and space elements.

§**"Pitta"**ayurvedic body type consist offire and water elements.

§

§ **"Kapha"** ayurvedic body type comprise of earth and the water elements.

Due to this reason the treatment to be followed in ayurveda for any ailment or disease be it chronic or some common problems need to be treated as per the body type of a person.

The charakasamhita and the susrutasamhita are the guide books of ayurvedic medicine which elaborate upon some eight branches in the study of ayurvedic medicine. The eight components of the branches of ayurveda are as follows:

1.Kayacikitsa or the internal medicine

2.2.Kaumarabhrtyam or Peaediatrics

3.3.Salya cikitsa or surgery

4.4.Salya tantra or eye

5.5.ENT Psychiatry or in Sanskrit – Bhutavidya

6.6.Agadatantram or toxicology

7.7. Rasayana or rejuvenation (Preventing diseases and improving immunity with rejuvenation)

8.8.Vajikaranam

For treatments ayurveda even uses animal products and minerals.

Is it safe to get medication from ayurvedic medicines?

Being the oldest form of treating ailments ayurveda, its effectiveness has been proven time and again. There have been testsupon the medicines used in ayurvedic medicines.Few of the tests conducted, concluded that in almost 40 percentage of some of the ayurvedic medicines contained elements such as arsenic.

However, the healthcare benefits of ayurveda have been in manifold in the past centuries.

Disadvantages of ayurvedic medicines:

It takes time to cure disease as per ayurveda.It is not like the allopathic medicines which work and show their effects. In ayurveda some medicinal preparation work fast some others take a lot of time to show their real effect. Treating diseases through ayurvedic medicines can in some case cause a burn in your pocket too!

Chapter 14: Balancing Vata Doşa Will Balance All Three Doşas

We can all keep ourselves healthily by simply balancing vata doşa, so the theory says. The general principles, by which vata doşa is to be balanced, are regularity and moderation.

Regularity

Regularity will mean sticking to a routine. This means that to stay in a condition of health, we must go to bed at the same time every day, arise at the same time every day, eat at the same time every day. Our shopping ought to be at the same time and place every week, and the same with our visiting or receiving visitors.

Can there be variety? Sure. As long as the variety doesn't exceed the regularity, then it is in balance and we can be healthy.

Moderation

Moderation means not too much of something, and being able to include every need. We must eat just enough and stop while we are still hungry, sleep only just enough, break up our working time with many short rests; ten minutes of resting after fifty minutes of working is a good amount.

Resting our eyes is also important. Whenever we are doing close work, such as reading or craft work with our hands on a table, for example, we need to take five minutes to look at a distance, at the end of every thirty minute session.

We must work only moderate amount of time per day, and also play, a moderate amount. Pleasure only a moderate amount. This is if we desire to be healthy.

How to Sleep

Scientific studies have shown that sleeping is twice as effective before astronomical midnight, as the sleep that is done after midnight. This means that whenever we sleep before midnight, then we need only half as many hours of sleep.

If our sleep is to be effective, we will have to lay ourselves down in perfect darkness, for any amount of light will interfere with the production of our sleep endorphins. For effective sleep, we must have excreted all the caffeine that we consumed in the previous day.

Good sleep requires that our bloodstream have in it no caffeine.

If you are having difficulty in getting to sleep, check out my booklet, "How to Sleep".

It is healthy to be asleep at midnight, and to be awake from 48 minutes before Sun's rising, and until the stars appear in the west at night. In special cases, a siesta during the day, after Sun has passed the meridian, is helpful. Still, it is preferable for this to be done in perfect darkness.

Sometimes one particular organ can need more prana. At a particular time of day, it makes one sleepy, not because of needing sleep, but because that organ needs more energy, or else it must be rested.

For example, people, who need to strengthen their stomachs, become sleepy between Sunrise and about 11:00 a.m.. This is no matter how much sleep they may have already had. But if they strengthen their stomachs, then they don't become sleepy at that time.

Principles of eating

If you follow this principle, then you will never get a cold nor flu.Consider 2 categories of food:

1)Animal foods, chemical additives, chemical medicines, alcohol, grains and sweets

2)Vegetables that grow above ground, and fruits

If your intaking of category 2 above is 2-3 times the amount of category 1, then you are unlikely to ever get cold or flu.

Do not mix fruits in your stomach with non-fruits.If you do, then the digestion fails, the byproducts rot, and it is worse than if you had not eaten them at all.

Ideally, melons and citrus fruits ought to each be in your stomach separately from each other and from all other foods.

Whole grains and beans together form a very good basis of one's diet, and supply all of the essential amino acids, plus needed calcium and magnesium.

Getting enough calcium and magnesium prevents chronic and degenerative diseases of all kinds, such as diabetes, heart disease, kidney stones, and arthritis.

Eat whole grains and not refined flour.Refined flour produces free radicals, and consequent deterioration of all organs.Anti-oxidants neutralize free radicals. Legumes are the most potent anti-oxidants.

Awakening and first routine of the day

Remember I told you that ayurveda is always in a state of development? The Dharma S'astras say that if you are Brahmana or Ksatriyya, and you have not the opportunity to support yourself through your proper method of livelihood, then you ought to resort to trade. The same is true of Sudras.

It is further suggested that you learn the art of trade from Vaisyas, that is to say from businessmen.

The most modern of businessmen recommend, as indispensable to proper success, that, if you are in business, you begin your day by reading at least 15 minutes from the scriptures, and 15 minutes from "motivational and success" books.

Any business teacher, who has himself become wealthy in business, ought to be able to give to you a list of these "motivational and success" books.

Daily routine

Here is an ayurvedic daily routine. There are variants for each of the 3 doşa types.

Awakening– The best time, for you to arise, depends upon your doşa type:

Vata type – 48 minutes before Sunrise. The 48 minute time measurement is called a "muhurtha."

The 48 minutes before Sunrise are the holiest time of the day, and are accordingly called the "Brahma Muhurtha."

Pitta type – One hour and 18 minutes before Sunrise.

Kapha type – Two hours and 18 minutes before Sunrise.

For people who have difficulty arising, I have given easy strategies to make it easier for you to awaken, and to remain awake, in my booklet, "Blueprint for A Super-Healthy (And Fun) Natural

Lifestyle."

Relax– The first thing we should do, upon awakening, is to relax. Preferably, this means performing the sāvāsana before arising from our bed.

Pray– Before you emerge from your bed of rest, ayurvedic sources recommend that you say a prayer

1. Affirming to God that he is inside of you and within your breath,

2. Requesting that compassion, love, peace, and joy be part of your life, and of all the people in your environs, in the coming day, and

3. That you be a healer, and that you be healed.

However, I must aver that if you have received The Knowledge of inner peace from Maharaji, which is the same as the s'astras call "knowing Brahman," then, instead of praying, you would do the techniques of The Knowledge in your bed of rest before arising, and this will be more effective for you than would be any prayer.

Clean and purefy your field with water and movements

Apply cold water to your face.

Rinse your mouth with water.

Wash your eyes. You can do this either with cool water, with doşa-specific eyewashes, or with cool herbal teas, particularly those made from herbs of your own area. I give myself an eyebath by pouring the liquid into one eye, then blinking a few times, then repeating in the other eye.

Some prefer to use an eyedropper, and some an eye cup, which is a specially designed cup just for washing your eyes. God has given me so much plantain herb growing outside my door, that I use it frequently for my eyewash.

Herbs for eyewashes:

- Angelica
- Borage
- Chamomile
- Chickweed

- Elder
- Fennel
- Golden seal
- golden seal + burnt alum
- hyssop
- marsh mallow
- plantain
- rock rose
- rosemary
- sarsaparilla
- sassafras
- slippery elm
- squaw vine
- tansy
- white willow
- wintergreen
- witch hazel
- yellow dock

Dosages for herbal eyewashes –Here are some "universal dosages" for herbal teas in general.

Ideal dosages may vary from plant to plant, but unless you have more specific information about the plant(s) that you intend to use, you can use these dosages:

To make an infusion tea from dried roots, seeds, or bark, here are two recipes:

Small Quantity:

4 teaspoons of dried root, seed, or bark. The metric equivalent would be 19 grams.

2 cups of boiling water. The metric equivalent would be 474 milliliters.

Pour the 2 cups of boiling water over over the 4 teaspoons of dried root, seed, or bark.

Let it steep 10 minutes.

After 10 minutes, strain off a quarter of a cup of the tea, allow it to become cool, and use it to wash your eyes. (2 fluid ounces -- 60 milliliters).

Larger Quantity:

- ¾ cup of root. The metric equivalent would be 170 grams.
- 3 quarts of boiling water. The metric equivalent would be 2.84 liters.

Pour the 3 quarts of boiling water over over the ¾ cup of root.

Let it steep 10 minutes.

After 10 minutes, strain off a quarter of a cup of the tea, wait for it to become cool, and use it to wash your eyes (2 fluid ounces -- 60 milliliters). You can refrigerate the remainder, and pull out the amount you need for washing your eyes, upon your awakening each morning.

To make an infusion tea from leaves or flowers, here is the recipe:

- 1 ¼ cups of leaves or flowers. The metric equivalent would be 284 grams.
- 4 ½ quarts of boiling water. The metric equivalent would be 3.9 liters.

Pour the 4 ½ quarts of boiling water over over the 1 ¼ cups of leaves or flowers.

Let it steep until it becomes cool. Then you can refrigerate it, and bring out the amount you need upon your awakening, and allow it to rise to room's temperature before using it to wash your eyes.

Herbal eyewash formula: 1 teaspoon goldenseal, 2 heaping teaspoons boric acid powder, and half a teaspoon of myrrh; steep in a pint of boiling water, and strain it after it becomes cool.

Eyewash for all 3 doşascombined is a combination of 3 Indian fruits, called "triphala." This can be obtained online. Put ¼ teaspoon of triphala into 1 cup of water, boil it for ten minutes, then allow it to become cool before straining it and washing your eyes with it.

Eyewash for pitta doşacan be cool water by itself. Alternatively, you can use rose water made from the petals of organically grown roses. Other type rose water you can buy might have chemicaux in the petals of the roses. The chemicaux sting the eyes, and are not beneficial as we would like them to be.

Eyewash for kapha doşais a mixture of from 3 to 5 drops of cranberry juice mixed into a teaspoon of distilled water. Mark you well, the store-boughten cranberry juice is likely to have in it sweeteners, city water, or other additives, so that is not the cranberry juice that we are looking for. Read the label before buying.

Then drink a glass of water, about 8 ounces, or ¼ liter. If you pour the water into a pure copper cup the night before, it will evacuate your kidneys, cause peristaltic motion to move matter through your

gastrointestinal tract, and it will wash more effectively your tract.

Best to leave off coffee and tea. Both of them are deleterious in that they are addictive, constipating, drain the adrenal glands, and take energy away from your kidneys, unless you leave off them.

Moreover, non-organically grown coffee is rich in heavy metal poisons.

Defecate– Ideally you would not put your feces into water, but in earth. If you use a public toilet, acquiring the skill of squatting on a toilet helps to save paper, and to prevent contact with the surface of the toilet. Squatting is inherently a better way to defecate, apart from the asepsis it creates.

After this becomes a regular habit for you, if you supped the night before, and yet cannot defecate, yet you are in healthy condition, some attention may be needed to your quality of sleep, or your digestive power.

Breathing from alternate nostrils in some cases induces movement of the bowels.

Both ayurveda, and the S'astras, enjoin you to use water to wash your anus after you defecate, using warm water, then to wash your hands using soap.

Tongue Dhauti -- This means gently scraping the top and sides of your tongue with an instrument. I use an upside-sown spoon. Yogis in India use a specially designed piece of wood.

Ayurvedic literature prescribes a different material for each person according to the doşa-type of their body. A scraper of gold is prescribed for the vata-type person, one of silver for the pitta-person, and of copper for the kapha-person.

In modern ayurvedic literature, stainless steel may be used by anybody.

As a guideline, or a rule-of-thumb, scrape your tongue 7-14 strokes from back to front, then from right to left, then from left to right, or vice-versa. Or do it until the spoon or scraper comes clean after a

stroke.

There are nerves and meridians in the tongue, which are favorably stimulated by this process, improving the health of your viscera.

Your digestion is thus improved.

Your tongue absorbs praṇa from food, by Jiminy. This is a great reason for you to keep it clean, because praṇa is going to give to you the health and the feeling that you would enjoy experiencing!

Another benefit of tongue-dhauti is the clearing of the way to the taste buds. The more taste you can sense from your food, the more saliva you will produce, and the better will your entire digestive tract

function.

The more saliva you produce, the more thoroughly your food will be utilized; moreover, your body is alkalinized by saliva, and that makes you immune to infectious diseases, such as anthrax, flu, colds, and all of them. The more alkaline your body, the more immune that you are.

A yogi suggests that you stick out your tongue and see how pretty it now looks, after you clean it.

Clean your teeth

- Your brush should be a soft one.
- Paste or powder ought to be bitter, pungent, and astringent.
- Indians have been in the habit of using neem sticks to brush their teeth. Besides removing particles from between the teeth, neem sticks also strengthen your gums, and assist them in being healthy.

Indians have also used licorice roots as toothbrushes.

- If your type is either kapha or vata, then a powder, made from almond shells roasted, is recommended.
- If your type is pitta, then ground neem powder is recommended.

My belief is that any fertile area of Earth will supply you with sticks and powders for cleaning your teeth, so that products needn't be imported from India or other places. This idea requires investigation by intuitive people who are in tune with both natural health, and also the Plant Kingdom.

Chapter 15: Sparshan Pareeksha- By Heartbeat Analysis (An Overview)

The established method for heartbeat examination among the Vaidya or Ayurvedic Practitioners is in indistinguishable way from it was hundreds of years prior. Pulse is analyzed by holding the hand by left hand for support.

The right hand's three fingertips, first, center and third finger, are kept somewhat pushed on the spiral heartbeat at Radial Fossa. The throbbing idea of the beat is watched rationally by the doctor. Vata is seen from the principal (distal or list) fingertip, Pitta is seen from the second (center) fingertip, Kaphha is seen from the third (proximal or ring) fingertip.

In the event that the debilitated individual is influenced by an abundance of Vata Dosha, the throbbing of heartbeat will be all the more effectively felt beneath the tip of first finger. In the event that the patient is experiencing the pitta dosha, the throbbing of the beat will be felt underneath the tip of the Middle finger, if thethrobbing of the beat is felt under the third finger, kapha dosha is watched.

In the event that throbbing of the beat is felt underneath the first and second finger, it implies the patient is experiencing the consolidated two doshas. In the event that throbbing of Pulse is felt under the first and third fingertip, it implies the debilitated is influenced from Vata and Kaphha Dosha.

In the event that the throbbing heartbeat is felt underneath the tip of second and third finger, which implies the patient is experiencing the Pitta and Kaphha Dosha. In the event that throbbing is felt beneath every one of the three fingertips that implies the patient is experiencing each of the three doshas, which is additionally called sannipat dosha.

The Doshas are changing inside the periods of life. Youth (0-16 Years) is ruled by an aggravation of Kapha, while grown-ups (16-50 Years) are confronting an unsettling influence of Pitta and older individuals (more than 50) an aggravation of Vata. These three stages apply as a rule.

Vata type

This dosha is made out of the Akasha and Vayu components and will in general be thin (lightest of the three body types) with cool dry skin and dry hair. They rush to get a handle on new thoughts, yet in addition rapidly to overlook. Vatas are described by eccentrics, energy, and inconstancy in eating regimen and rest. They tend tohave high vitality in short blasts yet tire effectively and over apply.

Vatas are inclined to cerebral pains, hypertension, nervousness, dry hacks, sore throats, ear infections, a sleeping disorder, unpredictable heart rhythms, premenstrual disorder, stomach gas, the runs, apprehensive stomach, clogging, muscle fits, bring down back agony, sexual dysfunctions, joint pain and sensory system issues.

Pitta type

Pitta types are made of Teja and Apa, are as a rule of medium form and quality, and can undoubtedly keep up their weight. They will in general be extreme, irascible, sharp-witted, energetic, have solid absorption, and a solid hunger. Pittas are methodical, effective, emphatic, and fearless, yet can end up forceful, requesting and pushy. They are genuinely unsurprising in their schedules as they eat three suppers per day and rest eight hours per night. By and large, their composition is reasonable or ruddy, regularly having spots, and their hair is generally fine and straight, inclining toward fair or red.

Common medical issues incorporate acid reflux, ulcers, hot sensations in the stomach or digestion tracts, a sleeping disorder, rashes or aggravations of the skin, skin inflammation, skin malignant growth, frailty, and gallbladder and liver issue.

Kapha type

Kapha people are made of strong, solid, overwhelming body type, and delicate hair and skin, for the most part with substantial delicate eyes and a low, delicate voice. They will in general put on weight effectively and require a great deal of rest and warmth. Kaphas are normally loose, elegant, moderate moving and friendly. They are pardoning, sympathetic, nonjudgmental, and steadfast. This dosha type has the most vitality of the considerable number of constitutions, yet it is relentless and persisting, not touchy.

Despite the fact that Kaphas for the most part have a solid protection from sickness, they are inclined to corpulence, sensitivities, colds, clog, sinus migraines, respiratory issues, atherosclerosis, and difficult joints.

What are the methods of Ayurvedic treatment?

There exists eight divisions of Ayurvedic therapeutics, to be specific Kayachikitsa (Internal solution), Shalya (Surgery), Shalkya (Otorhinolaryngology and Opthalmology), Kaumr Bhritya (Pediatrics, Gynecology and Obstetrics) Agad tantra (Toxicology), Rasayana (Gerentorology), Vajikaran (Aphrodisiacs) and Bhoot Vidya (Psychiatry).

The standards of treatment are Shodhan (purificatory), Shaman (palliative and moderate), Nidan parivarjan (shirking of causative and prescipitating components of malady) and Pathya Vyavastha (do's and don'ts with respect to weight control plans way of life). Shodhan treatment incorporates Vamana (therapeutically initiated emesis), Virechana (restoratively prompted laxation), Vasti (cured douche), shirovirechana (organization of pharmaceuticals through nose) and Raktmokshan (Blood letting). These remedial techniques are all things considered known as Panchkarma. Before executing Panchkarma treatment Snehan (olation) and Swedan (getting sweat) are to utilized first.

Does Ayurvedic arrangement of solution have in addition to focuses over traditional restorative framework?

Being comprehensive and sickness eradicative with standards of individualized treatment, conducive to financial states of India and with accessibility of plenitude of details for a specific malady, utilization of food things as solution and way of life tenets, Ayurveda appreciates a superior place in regard of counteractive action and cure of the illness is worried in contrast with western medicinal framework.

Could one bring Ayurveda Medicine with present day pharmaceuticals?

If not demonstrated generally by the going to doctor, Ayurveda Medicines can by and large be taken along with allopathic pharmaceuticals. Also, Ayurveda Medicines are utilized as adjuvant to allopathic pharmaceuticals in the vast majority of perpetual and degenerative maladies. In that capacity there is no damage to devour straightforward home grown plans of Ayurveda even without the remedy of the specialist yet mineral based meds must be utilized after due conference and counsel of the specialist.

What are the basic Ayurveda Medicines which can be utilized without counseling the specialists?

Straightforward natural medications like powders, pills and tablets, syrups and decoctions can be utilized for the administration of basic illnesses like hack, chilly, fever, acid reflux, spewing, the runs, loss of craving, body and joint agonies and so forth, even without the solution of a specialist. Correspondingly, natural tonics/wellbeing food can likewise be devoured if the same don't make any disturbing distress or surprises.

Rasayana

"Rasayana" comprise of two words "Rasa" and "Ayana". "Rasa" implies embodiment of something. Anything indigested into the body as food or pharmaceutical initially is incorporated into Rasa Dhatu; the fundamental plasma tissue. Ayana is the technique by which "Rasa" is conveyed to all body tissues for biochemical transformation. So "Rasayana" implies what decimates the maturity and sickness through the preservation, change and renewal of vitality. This revival treatment involves a remarkable position in study of Ayurveda. It keeps the body youthful and lithe even after one has passed his or her childhood.

What is Rasayana?

Admission of Anti Aging Herbs (that are Rasayana in Ayurveda) In Ayurveda hostile to maturing can likewise be comprehended as far as RASAYANAA: and it is said in Ayurveda that what makes new again or reestablishes ones young condition of physical and psychological wellness and also grow our condition of bliss.

The word Rasayanaa, i.e. rasa + ayana alludes to food and its transportation in the body. Such a condition of enhanced nourishment is asserted to prompt a progression of auxiliary properties like aversion of maturing and life span, resistance against maladies, mental skill and expanded imperativeness of the body.

'Rasa', the exacting importance of Rasa is the substance of our food after absorption, first Rasa Dhatu (Chyle) shapes, Ayan implies way or way.

Accordingly, just the element which increment Rasa Dhatu and sustains all the seven Dhatus is called Rasayana. Along these lines, in helpful process Rasa is worried with the protection, change, and renewal of vitality. Rasa sustains our body, supports invulnerability and keeps the body and psyche in the best of wellbeing.

Aversion and administration of these medical issues could help the elderly to enhance personal satisfaction and stay self –dependent for their every day exercises to most extreme conceivable degree. Ayurveda has an engaged branch called Rasayana (rejuvenation) which manages the issues identified with maturing and strategies to counter the same. Rasayana treatment gives higher imperviousness to infections, brings serenity, de-push the psyche calming it from uneasiness, sadness and stress related issues.

Different advantages of Rasayana treatment are:-

Long Life

Increase memory

Good wellbeing

Young looks

Glowing skin

Calmness

Resistance to infection

As we as a whole know the Rasayana treatment being a piece of Ayurveda is absolutely a Herbal Treatment and along these lines can without much of a stretch be suggested for pregnant ladies, kids, elderly or the individuals who are incapacitated, anorexic, convalescents, for pallor and Vata conditions.

Vajikarna

Vajikarana is the name given for Ayurvedic aphrodisiacs. They not just lift up the sex wellbeing; they additionally tone up the genital framework. It furnishes torque with a point of view of sexual execution. Vajikarana is both a Swasthasya urjaskara (reestablishing wellbeing in effectively sound people) and Artasya Roganut (malady reducing and changing kind of solutions). They advance physical and psychological well-being. They can be promptly utilized as a part of treating Premature Ejaculation.

Ahara (food), Nidra (Sleep) and Brahmacharya (Celibacy) are the tripod of our life. They should be adjusted regarding quality and amount for the duration of our life to ensure that they are organizing with each other and furthermore helping us live soundly. For this we have to have a restrained existence. We require all those 3, yet there is a period and strategy to devour them.

Advantages of Rasayana and Vajikarna in mental problems

We as a whole need to look youthful and feel enthusiastic constantly. Maturing, being a characteristic procedure can't be ceased yet it can be deferred by taking after a sound way of life. Ayurveda gives us hostile to maturing tips that help us to know the successful approaches to back off the maturing procedure. There are old treatments and present day medications that adequately diminish the impacts of maturing.

- Aging is a characteristic procedure
- It is a nonstop procedure
- It increments with time
- It can't be ceased yet can be backed off

A cell may supplant itself with a weaker cell each time. A cell will do this on the off chance that it hasn't had the privilege nutritious nourishments accessible to it. This procedure is called degeneration.

A cell can supplant itself with a similar quality cell. This implies the body doesn't make strides. That is, you have an interminable condition. The cell is equipped for supplanting itself with a more grounded and better cell. This will happen just if the cell has a plenitude of vitality and the correct crude materials. This procedure is called recovery. This is hostile to maturing.

Panchkarma: Your Best Detoxification

It's called Panchkarma and signifies "five activities." The advantages of this old, altogether normal Detox technique are being re-found today. This arrangement of methods was first portrayed in the antiquated records of Ayurveda. A quote from the Charaka Samhita, one of the old established writings of Ayurvedic instructing (around 400 BC), depicts the fundamentals of this capable Detox device:

"In a man whose stomach related framework has been washed down and sanitized the digestion is invigorated, illness is decreased, and typical wellbeing is kept up. Sense organs, psyche, astuteness and composition are enhanced; quality, great support, sound descendants and power are the outcome. Manifestations of maturing don't show up so effortlessly and the individual lives long and free from scatters. Consequently, end treatment ought to be done accurately and at the correct time."

Panchkarma treatment is a genuinely extraordinary approach for renewal, revival and counteractive action. Legitimate Ayurvedic Detox is not done piecemeal. The medicines are proposed to be done in cautious succession, not in segregation. Each stage and step, physiologically, bolsters the following. This is one sign of "valid" imperial Panchkarma: the medicines are executed as endorsed by the writings — in a bona fide way — enabling the most extreme advantage to be inferred. What takes after is a preliminary for understanding true Panchkarma, from, Ayurveda, and your best Detox.

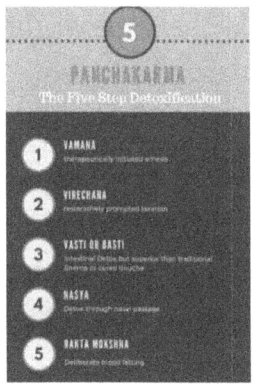

1. Vamana: The process of inducing vomiting, to eliminate the impurities from the body is known as Vamana. This deliberate vomiting is employed to treat, aggravated Kapha. Vamana is indicated in the treatment of anorexia, bronchial

asthma, cough, diabetes mellitus, epilepsy, goiter, obesity and Urticaria.

2. Virecahna: The process of inducing purgation to eliminate the impurities from the body (Detox) is known as Virechana. It is done in disease caused by the aggravation of Pitta. Virechana treatment is useful in the disease like arthritis, asthma, constipation, intestinal disorders, jaundice, piles, seminal-diseases, skin-diseases, enlarged spleen, and worm infestation.

3. Vasti or Basti is the process of inducing herbal oils in the intestines through anal, urinary and vaginal region. It considered as the main and superior treatment among five stages of Panchkarma. According to Ayurvedic practice, vasti has capability to cure severe diseases. Vasti is administered in abdominal distension, arthritis, cervical-spondylosis, constipation, emaciation, enlarged spleen, facial paralysis, headache, hemiplegia, lumbar-spondylosis and urinary retention.

4. Nasya is the process of inducing medicated oils in the nasal passage for the treatment of diseases above the neck. Nasya is very efficacious in the treatment of upper respiratory tract diseases, allergic rhinitis, hay fever, migraine, frontal sinusitis, atrophic rhinitis, epilepsy and viral catarrh.

5. Rakta Mokshana is process of deliberate bloodletting. It is rarely used these days.

It is used in curing diseases caused by aggravation of blood. Blood is important tissue (dhatu) of the human body and is involved in many diseases.

Other procedure used for detoxification in Ayurveda

Abhyanga

Abhyanga is the name of the synchronized oil treatment, changed in accordance with every person. Amid Abhyanga two advisors tenderly treat the patient at the same time, in a set way. Women are dealt with by female specialists; men by male advisors. Abhyanga ousts from the body tissues those poisons and waste items that have as of now been broken down by the before methodology. Abhyanga is done peacefully, which blends the body's capacities. Hush and rest are essential parts during the time spent enacting the body's own particular self-mending instruments. The abhyanga treatment utilizes home grown substances and decision fixings uniquely set up together for the individual patient. These fixings are arranged together with alleviating oils, in our own particular oil kitchen.

Vishesh

This is a full-body treatment completed by two specialists applying additional weight. It serves to unwind the muscles significantly, and intensely animates the flow in the tissues.

Garshan

An activity with crude silk gloves making erosion on the surface of the skin and expanding flow in the body. It advances weight reduction and cleans up stopping up debasements that may bring about issues, for example, cellulite. Garshan is trailed by oil treatment.

Udvarthana

This treatment with glue made with ground grains and natural powders washes down the skin, builds dissemination and backings sound weight.

Pizhichill

Pizhichill is an exceptional type of treatment, somewhere between oil treatment and warmth treatment. In this alleged "imperial treatment" a tender, synchronized activity is done under a consistent stream of warm home grown oil. This treatment is exceedingly valued by all visitors and delivers great outcomes supporting joint wellbeing and mitigating muscle strain.

Svedana

The oil treatment is regularly trailed by a home grown steam shower with extraordinarily chose restorative herbs. This expands the vessels and subsequently helps the detoxification of the framework. The term Svedana incorporates a wide range of types of warmth treatment. The warmth can be dry or sodden, connected locally or to the entire body.

Basti

Toward the finish of every day, after the polluting influences from various parts of the body have been extricated and drawn into the intestinal tract, the patient gets a basti. These delicate interior purifying medications utilize either warm herbalised oil or water-based home grown decoctions to wipe out polluting influences from the intestinal tract. This is a standout amongst the most critical parts of treatment; as per the old Ayurvedic writings "with basti alone half of sickness can be diminished."

Shirodhara

An unwinding treatment to the head, in which a flood of warm oil streams equitably over the temple, going on for quite a while. Shirodhara treatment is done in outright quiet, prompting profound unwinding and an adjusted condition of rest at the top of the priority list and body. Men and ladies alike experience it as a high purpose of Panchakarma applications.

Nasya

Nasya underpins solid sinuses, quiets bothered memory and backings ordinary hearing capacity (e.g. tinnitus). Careful medicines to the head, shoulders and neck, inward breaths and packs are the all around adjusted procedures of this profoundly compelling treatment. An extra advantage of nasya treatment, as indicated by Ayurveda, is that it is said to fortify the brain and astuteness.

Netra Tarpana

Today's reality is immersed with visual incitement. Our eyes can be stressed and abused, which can make an unfriendly impact on our vision and cerebrum action. Netra tarpana treatment relaxingly affects the eyes and encompassing tissue. It is completed in conjunction with the use of home grown oil to the face and is experienced by customers as extremely charming and unwinding.

Pinda Sveda

Little cloth sacks loaded with uncommonly arranged home grown blends are connected locally to alleviate torment. An extra real part in this treatment is played by the exceptionally effective Ayurveda home grown oils which are extraordinarily chosen by the specialist for the parts of the body that are difficult. The impact of the natural concentrates is to ease the agony, and to unwind and develop the influenced zone.

The Concept of Sattva

Sattva

Sattva is a pseudo Dosha as it is without any evil character. Numerous Ayurveda specialists don't think of it as a Dosha as Dosha is an equivalent word of polluting influence or sick quality. Sattva is otherwise called 'Mahaguna" which signifies "the super quality ". In spite of the fact that it is a mind boggling subject, Sattva can be extensively accepted as something;

- Spiritual
- Close to the god
- Perfection
- Noble
- Calm
- Good for body and brain
- Good signals and Habits

As indicated by the Vedic science, the entire universe is comprised of five fundamental components;

1. Air
2. Earth
3. Sky
4. Fire
5. Water

What's more, three Mahagunas:

- Sattva
- Rajas
- Tamas

Qualities of Sattva

Every one of the general population with various identity qualities have diverse dimension of Mahaguna: Sattva, Rajas and Tamas in them. A honorable man would have a high extent of Sattva and low extent of rajas and Tamas. Thus a ravenous individual would have low Sattva, high Rajas and Tamas. An individual with criminal mindset would have low Sattva, low Rajas and High Tamas.

Attributes (Prakurti) of a High Sattva individual:

- Individual who is holy person.
- Have a decent heart.
- Does philanthropy work.
- Noble soul.
- Intellectual, astute.

- Peaceful.
- Sharp memory.
- Calm.
- have an unlimited authority on self feelings and conduct.
- Law standing.
- Socially regarded.
- Simple living and high reasoning.
- Devoid of adoration for the materialistic things.
- Prefers cotton or silk fiber garments which are normal and non extravagant.
- listens profound and great music.
- reads profound books and shows the leanings to other people.
- is a genuine master.

Qualities of high Sattva nourishment

Food which are:

- Sweet
- Fresh
- Juices

- Energy giving
- Easily edible
- Fruits and vegetables
- Milk
- Wheat
- Cucumber
- Nuts
- Nutritious Food, that is useful for body and soul

Everybody should endeavor to include Sattva characteristics throughout their life. This is an ordinary learning and Sattva is a learning quality. Otherworldliness is an incredible method to grasp Sattva properties in the life. Essentially we have distinguished the Sattva properties and need to simply include each Sattva characteristics throughout your life and decline the Rajas and Tamas attributes.

Aachaar Rasayana and Sadvrataa (Code of lead) - The pathway to Sattva

The master's from the Vedic time frame have portrayed the Sadvrataa to get the most astounding emotional well-being and to establish a framework of a superior society. In the Various Ayurveda Samhitas(Literature) there has been depicted some Sadvrataa guidelines to be pursued for the Rasayana course which are called Aachar Rasayana. It originates from the word Aachar(behavior, character ,direct) + Rasayana. The proposals Described under Aachar Rasayana are additionally useful in keeping up mental and social wellbeing simply like Sadvrataa. Counting trhese into Rasayana indicates that:

1.Practicing Sadvrataa(Code of lead) is useful for psychological well-being just as social wellbeing and furthermore increment the essential impact of Rasayana in the body. The mind impacts the body.

2.Without rehearsing the Sadvrataa, Rasayana is of no utilization.

Rehearsing the sadvritta(Code of lead) keeps up an abnormal state of Sattva in the psyche and it checks the dimension of Rajas and Tamas. This don't give any mental sickness a chance to develop in the brain.

Chapter 16: Ashwaganda

Withania somnifera, widely known as Ashwagandha (winter cherry), is an important medicinal plant that has been used for more than 3,000 years in Ayurvedic and Indigenous medicine. Some herbalists refer to the Indian ginseng as Ashwagandha. The plant extract has several bioactive compounds and therefore performs antioxidant, anti-inflammatory, and immunomodulating activities. The plant bioactive compounds and its extract are used in the treatment and prevention of many diseases, including arthritis, impotence, amnesia, anxiety, cancer, cardiovascular and neurodegenerative disorders, among others. This chapter discusses Ashwagandha's various health benefits in both humans and animals.

Ashwagandha's top surprising health benefits

It helps manage weight gain and diminish eating comfort.

This powerful herb often helps to control body weight when stress is an issue. Psychological stress is often linked to weight gain and obesity since increased levels of stress hormones can lead to increased weight gain over long periods. Chronic stress can also lead to changes in eating behavior- the comfort of eating and reaching for biscuit tin in the face of pressure is all too easy. Ashwagandha can be used in adults under chronic stress for bodyweight management, helping them to minimize the effects of stress on bad food cravings, and to maintain more physical activity.

It improves both sexual performance and libido.

Ashwagandha is traditionally used both for men and women to improve sexual performance and libido. We produce a lot more adrenaline when we are stressed and put pressure on our adrenal glands and organs. Ashwagandha regulates the quantity of adrenaline released and strengthens the organs, improves stamina, increases sperm count and motility in men, and improves libido among women. One study showed that women who had taken a daily dose of Ashwagandha over a month saw significant improvements in achieving orgasm and sexual arousal as a result of a substantial reduction in sexual distress. In addition to decreasing the effects of stress, it was suggested that the role of Ashwagandha in increasing testosterone was also crucial as this is a factor in the syndrome of androgen deficiency, which is also associated with female sexual dysfunction.

Supports brain function and memory.

Also of growing importance impact on brain function, including memory. Naturally, Ashwagandha has been used to boost memory in Ayurveda, which is evaluated to encourage antioxidant exercise, which guards nerve cells toward destructive free radicals. Healthy men who regularly took Ashwagandha showed substantial improvements in their reaction time and task performance in one study compared to men who got a placebo. Another 8-week research in 50 adults found that taking 300 mg of ashwagandha root extract twice daily greatly improved overall memory, the efficiency of the operations, and attention.

Making immunity greater.

Most adaptogenic herbs affect our immune system positively, and Ashwagandha is no exception. Traditionally, it is used to support a weakened immune system, and it has now been demonstrated to inspire anti-inflammatory and disease-fighting immune cells that help avoid disease. More work is required, but early studies are promising, such as one showing a significant change in the activation of immune cells after taking Ashwagandha. In that context, Ashwagandha can be used during treatments such as chemotherapy or radiotherapy to help the immune system.

Conclusion

Ayurveda is a traditional method to treat different heath problems with herbal ingredients. These products are safe to detoxify your body and cure any disease. The Ayurveda practitioner will examine your body to determine your basic dosha and check the balance among all three doshas. The practitioner will examine your stools, urine and check your body weight. Feel your pulse because every dosha creates a particular pulse. Listen to your voice and speech and look at your skin, tongue, teeth and eyes.

Your Ayurveda treatment will depend on your primary dosha, balance between these doshas and unique prakriti. They try to clean undigested food from your body and this cleansing procedure is known as panchakrama. This procedure may include blood purification, medical oils through nose, massage, vomiting and use of laxatives, enemas or purgatives to purify your intestines. If you want to treat your body with the help of Ayurveda medication, you can use herbal products to make your own medicine.

www.ingramcontent.com/pod-product-compliance
Lightning Source LLC
Chambersburg PA
CBHW071446070526
44578CB00001B/238